Practical
Equine
Dermatology

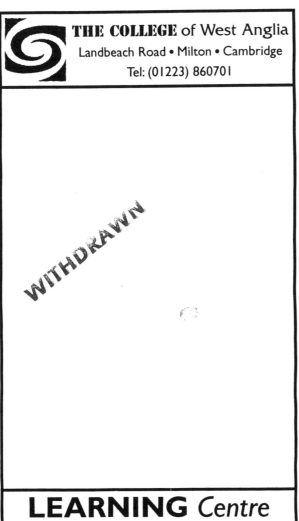

Practical Equine Dermatology

D. H. Lloyd, J. D. Littlewood,
J. M. Craig and L. R. Thomsett

Blackwell
Science

Published by Blackwell Science, a Blackwell Publishing company
Editorial offices:
Blackwell Science Ltd, 9600 Garsington Road, Oxford OX4 2DQ, UK
    Tel: +44 (0) 1865 776868
Iowa State Press, a Blackwell Publishing Company, 2121 State Avenue, Ames,
Iowa 50014-8300, USA
    Tel: +1 515 292 0140
Blackwell Science Asia Pty, 550 Swanston Street, Carlton, Victoria 3053,
Australia
    Tel: +61 (0)3 8359 1011

First published 2003

Library of Congress Cataloging-in-Publication Data
    p. cm.
Includes bibliographical references.
  ISBN 0-632-04807-7 (pbk. : alk. paper)
  1. Horses--Diseases. 2. Veterinary dermatology. I. Lloyd, D. H.
(David Hanbury)

  SF959.S54P73 2003
  636.1'08965--dc21   2003012192

ISBN 0-632-04807-7

A catalogue record for this title is available from the British Library

Set in Palatino and produced
by Gray Publishing, Tunbridge Wells, Kent
Printed and bound in Denmark using acid-free paper
by Narayana Press, Odder

For further information on Blackwell Publishing, visit our website:
www.blackwellpublishing.com

Contents

Preface   **vii**

Acknowledgements   viii

1   The diagnostic approach   **1**

Taking the history   1

Clinical examination   2

Diagnostic tests   3

2   Pruritus   **9**

Contagious conditions   9

Non-contagious conditions   17

3   Crusting and scaling   **25**

Seborrhoea   25

Idiopathic seborrhoea   25

Infectious causes   27

Bacterial infection   30

Viral infection   35

Immune-mediated causes   35

Environmental causes   40

Uncertain aetiology   42

4   Ulcers and erosions   **47**

Contagious causes   47

Congenital and hereditary causes   53

Environmental and nutritional causes   55

Neoplastic causes   57

Miscellaneous dermatoses   57

5	**Nodules and swellings**	**63**
	Physical conditions	64
	Infectious causes	66
	Fungal infections	77
	Parasitic infestations	80
	Neoplasia	83
	Immune-mediated causes	87
	Miscellaneous	88
	Cysts	93
6	**Coat problems**	**100**
	Alopecia	100
7	**Pigmentary disorders**	**109**
	Hypopigmentation – genetic or acquired	109
	Other pigmentary changes considered to be genetic in aetiology	111
	Hypopigmentation following inflammation	112
8	**The foot and associated structures**	**115**
	The hoof wall	115
	Examination of the foot	117
	Disorders of the foot	120
	Acquired disorders of the hoof	120
	The frog	122
	Neoplasia of the frog	124
	Necrosis	124
	The sole	125
9	**Therapy in equine dermatology**	**126**
	Availability of veterinary medicines for equine patients	126
Sources of drugs, topical products and instruments		**128**
References and further reading		**130**
Index		**133**

Preface

Equine practice has become increasingly sophisticated in recent years, at a time when horses are more numerous in the UK than they have ever been. Skin problems have always been common in the horse and often present the clinician with a challenge. The growing need for readily accessible and practical information on equine dermatology presented by modern equine and mixed veterinary practice provided the stimulus for this book.

The aim has been to provide a concise, problem-oriented, text facilitating a well-organised diagnostic approach together with a basic knowledge of dermatology in a practical format illustrated with pictures of the principal conditions, particularly those in which visual information is an important part of diagnosis. All of the conditions likely to be encountered in the UK are included and information on rarer conditions, such as those that may occur in imported horses, is also provided.

The book will be valuable to equine practitioners and those in mixed practice who see horses from time to time. Veterinary surgeons with an interest in the wider field of veterinary dermatology as well as undergraduates and postgraduate students will find the text useful as a key reference to skin problems of the horse.

This book is intentionally brief. A list of references is provided for further information on specific topics and also to direct the reader towards general texts with a wider range of information. The authors hope that this text will not only provide practical help on the everyday problems of skin disease in equine practice but that it will also stimulate a deeper interest in equine dermatology.

Indications for treatment are given within the text. Generally, these are based on UK practice and on products available within the UK. Where unlicensed preparations are mentioned readers should note that these are used only when licensed products are not available.

Descriptions of the use of unlicensed products or 'off label' use of licensed products have been italicised. Efficacy and safety of unlicensed products and 'off label' use cannot be guaranteed. Issues relating to drug use in horses are considered in the appendix.

David H. Lloyd
Janet D. Littlewood
J. Mark Craig
Lovell R. Thomsett

ACKNOWLEDGEMENTS

The authors would like to acknowledge the contributions of Mr Carl Temple, who drew the line drawings, and of Dr Cathy McGowan, who read the final draft and made many useful suggestions. Many of the illustrations were provided by colleagues; we relied on the Royal Veterinary College Dermatology Group slide collection and also wish to acknowledge in particular contributions from Dr Stephen Shaw, Mr Andrew Browning, Dr Keith Barnett, Dr Sandy Bjornson, Ms Pauline Williams, Dr Harriet Brooks, Dr Liz Steeves and Dr Malcolm Brearley.

DISCLAIMER

While every care has been taken by the authors and publisher to ensure that the drug uses, dosages and information in this book are accurate, errors may occur and readers should refer to the manufacturer or approved labelling information for additional information.

Readers should also note that this text includes information on drugs that are not licensed for use in horses. Readers should therefore check manufacturer's product information before using such drugs.

The diagnostic approach

A structured approach is essential. Vital information is usually obtained during the history taking process and sufficient time must be allowed for this. Accurate information on husbandry is particularly important. Clinical examination must include systemic and skin components. The process is illustrated with flow diagrams (Figures 1.1 and 1.2).

TAKING THE HISTORY

The approach (Figure 1.1) is similar to that adopted in other species. Points to include are:

- Breed, age and sex, origin. Consider these aspects carefully. In many conditions these simple data will have an important impact on your diagnostic considerations.
- Type of husbandry and use.
  - Length of time owned.
  - Feeding regimen.
  - Periods spent in stable or at pasture.
  - Type of stable and bedding; stable hygiene, contamination.
  - Conditions in paddocks.
  - Seasonal changes in management.
  - Routine management procedures, vaccination, deworming.
  - Grooming procedures; sharing of grooming kit, tack, grooms.
  - Equipment used in contact with the horse – boots, bandages and so on.
  - Use of horse – hunting, breeding, racing.
  - Contact with other horses, other species; opportunities for transmission of disease.

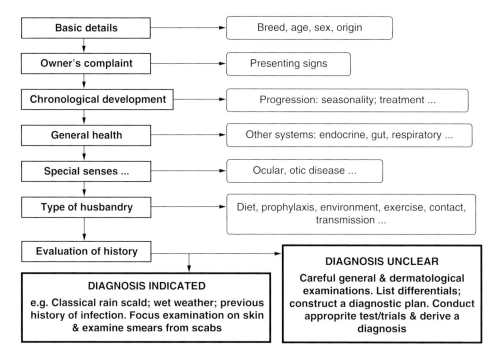

Figure 1.1   Taking the history. Components and the sequence of the history taking process. Analysis of the history should enable the clinician to construct an initial list of differential diagnoses that may help to focus the clinical examination along particular diagnostic lines. It may enable the diagnostic process to be abbreviated where a likely diagnosis is indicated or it may point towards the need for a more detailed approach.

- History of the current problem.
  - First signs, progression, response to treatment and management changes.
  - Seasonal effects.
  - Any diagnostic test results.
  - Current or recent therapy; include questions about use of unregistered remedies.
  - Previous episodes of disease.
  - Evidence of transmission; lesions in humans.
- General health.

CLINICAL EXAMINATION

A full clinical examination of both the general health status and the skin is necessary in most cases. Ensure that the animal is adequately restrained

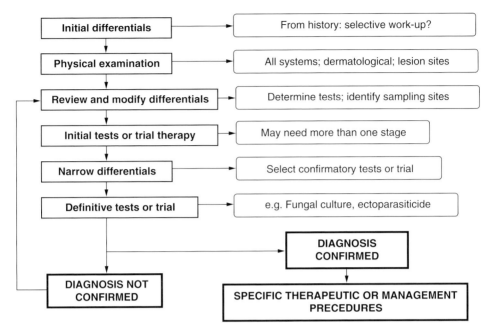

Figure 1.2 Clinical examination and diagnostic procedures. A thorough general and dermatological examination should be carried out unless the history points clearly towards a diagnosis. Examination coupled with history enable formulation of the diagnostic plan and the selection of appropriate tests and sites to be sampled, and/or therapeutic trials.

and you have sufficient light. Work systematically down each body region, beginning at the head and ending at the tail and perineal region. Be sure to include all aspects of the feet including the coronary band and the frog. You may need to clean the skin to observe some lesions. In some instances sedation may be necessary.

A record of the distribution and severity of primary and secondary lesions should be kept. Forms including a horse outline make this much easier.

It may be helpful to visit and examine the paddocks and exercise areas used.

DIAGNOSTIC TESTS

The history and clinical examination should enable you to formulate a list of differential diagnoses. It may help to create a problem list, identifying the predominant clinical signs, categorising them as contagious or non-contagious and allocating the disease within the following groups, which form the basis for the problem-orientated approach in this book: pruritic, crusting and scaling, ulcerative and erosive, nodular or swollen, alopecic; pigmentary; pedal.

A diagnostic plan can then be constructed, diagnostic procedures selected and samples collected. Sample collection may include the following techniques.

Hair plucks

Useful to determine whether the condition is pruritic (fractured hair shafts suggesting self-trauma) and to examine for dermatophytes and for parasite eggs.

- Choose a fresh, unmedicated lesion.
- For suspected dermatophytosis, where cultures are required, first lightly clean the areas to be sampled with 70% alcohol (to reduce contaminant organisms).
- Tissue or epilation forceps can be used to gently grasp and pull out any broken and intact hairs from the periphery of the lesion. Samples can be held in paper envelopes or sterile non-airtight universal containers pending examination.

Crusts

Useful for examination by bacterial (especially dermatophilosis) and fungal culture, and cytology.

- Choose a fresh, unmedicated lesion.
- Impression smears of the bases of freshly removed crusts, stained with Gram's stain or Giemsa can provide a quick method of diagnosis for dermatophilosis.
- Crusts can be collected and held in paper envelopes or sterile containers.

Tape strippings

This technique can be used to look for eggs (*Oxyuris equi*), ectoparasites and cutaneous microorganisms such as bacteria and yeasts.

- 3M Scotch tape is recommended for tape strippings.
- The tape is held between thumb and forefinger of both hands and pressed firmly against the area ensuring full contact of the adhesive surface with the affected skin.
- Mount the tape on a glass slide. For bacteria, fungi or cytology, stain with a rapid stain such as DiffQuik (Wardle Chemicals) and examine under the microscope.

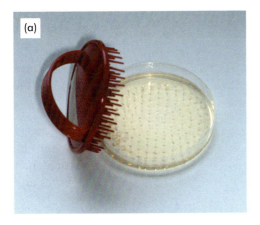
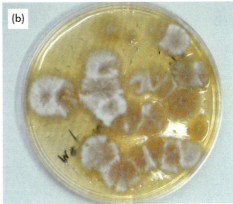

Figure 1.3 (a) A coarse-toothed brush (e.g. 90 mm Denman scalp brush) facilitates sampling of large areas of skin and coat. The collected hair can be removed and examined or the teeth may be embedded in a fungal culture medium as illustrated. (b) Here, *Microsporum canis* has been isolated using this technique.

Coat brushings

These allow for examination for dermatophytes and external ectoparasites where the lesions are diffuse or extensive. Scrapings are better for resident mite infestations.

- Use a sterile scalp brush (Mackenzie brush technique; Figure 1.3a and b), or toothbrush, to brush firmly over the lesions. Place the brush in an envelope or toothbrush tube to protect it prior to submission for dermatophyte culture.
- A scalp brush or tongue depressor can be used to brush directly into a sterile Petri dish, for mites, lice and other external parasites.

Skin scrapings

Skin scrapings can be performed for detection of external parasitic diseases such as chorioptic mange, larval stages of harvest mites, demodicosis (rare) or for dermatophyte culture and cytology.

- If there is excess hair over these areas, clip the hair carefully.
- Using a large, curved scalpel blade (e.g. number 22), lightly moisten the blade or area to be sampled with liquid paraffin (more useful for examination of mites), water or normal saline (for dermatophytes and mite examinations).
- Gently scrape the superficial crusts, scales and associated hair so that it accumulates on the blade. Mix the material with liquid paraffin,

water or saline (whichever was used on the skin) on a microscopic slide, apply a coverslip and examine under the microscope.
- Sample several suspect areas. Collect plenty of material and divide amongst several slides to make thin suspensions, which are quicker and easier to examine efficiently.
- Deeper scrapings need to be taken for suspected demodicosis. In this case the scraping should be deep enough to cause capillary ooze.
- For dermatophytes, clean the areas to be sampled lightly with 70% alcohol (to reduce the number of contaminating microbes).

Direct smears

From fresh exudative crusting, excoriated or pustular lesions, a direct impression smear can be made to enable examination of bacteria, fungi, protozoa and cytology.

- Press a glass slide against the concave undersurface of any plucked exudative crust, or against the surface of a freshly exposed lesion.
- For an intact pustule, gently break the skin covering the pustule with a 25 g needle and press a clean glass slide to it. Alternatively, the pus may be collected in the needle bevel or on a dry swab and then transferred to the glass slide.
- Air-dry and store the slide in a slide box prior to heat fixing (Gram's staining) or immersion in methanol for 5 min (for Giemsa or DiffQuik staining).

Swabs

May be useful for bacteriology and yeast or dermatophyte culture.

- If the sample is to be processed shortly after collection (c. 30 min), a dry sterile swab can be used for bacterial and fungal culture, and smears. Otherwise, use swabs with aerobic and anaerobic transport media.
- Samples collected from the skin surface are rarely representative of the causative agent, therefore collect pus from an intact pustule or underside of scab, or submit biopsy material.
- Biopsy specimens are more representative.

Needle aspirates

- A 20–22 g needle and 5–10 ml syringe can be used. The area to be aspirated should be carefully disinfected. The needle is inserted into the nodule (Figure 1.4) or mass and used to probe the tissue in several places whilst aspirating.

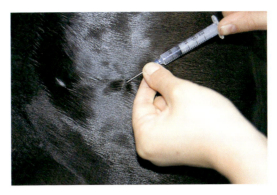

Figure 1.4   Fine needle aspiration of nodular lesions. (Courtesy of Liz Steeves.)

- The needle is withdrawn from the tissue and detached from the syringe. The syringe is then filled with air, reattached to the needle and the sample expelled directly onto a clean slide for cytology. Otherwise keep the sample in the needle and syringe until it can be transferred to a swab for culture.

Biopsy samples

The biopsy sample may be collected for a variety of reasons, e.g. histopathology, fungal or bacterial culture, viral identification with electron microscopy, immunohistochemistry. If in doubt, consult a pathologist as to the best way to process and transport the biopsy to the laboratory.

There are three common ways to take biopsy samples: by excision, shaving or biopsy punch (Figure 1.5). The most common is the punch technique described below.

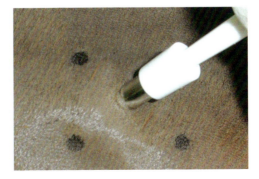

Figure 1.5   The punch biopsy procedure enables rapid sampling and is suitable for the majority of equine lesions. (Courtesy of Harriet Brooks.)

- It is generally necessary to sedate the horse. For sensitive areas especially on distal parts of limbs, a nerve block may be performed, e.g. low or high four point or abaxial sesamoid, depending on the area involved.
- Areas that include primary lesions and are not marred by chronicity or medication should be chosen. Take multiple biopsy samples unless only one lesion type and stage is present.
- Because sample orientation during histopathology cannot be predicted, ensure that the whole punch sample includes tissue of interest. If normal tissue is to be included this should be taken as a separate sample. Where you wish to investigate the transition between lesional and healthy skin, take an elliptical excision sample.
- The selected sites may be marked using a coloured marker. Try to avoid areas overlying superficial ligaments, blood vessels, nerves or superficial synovial structures associated with tendons and joints. It is important *not to prepare the site surgically before sampling.*
- The selected sites may be anaesthetised by injecting approximately 1–2 ml of lignocaine hydrochloride without adrenaline into the subcutaneous tissue below the lesions.
- Wait for 2–5 min and test the anaesthesia at the site with a needle.
- Use a 6–9 mm biopsy punch. Generally the larger punch is better. Ensure the blade is sharp.
- Once the punch is withdrawn, the biopsy sample may be attached to underlying structures by a thin attachment. Grasp the tissue sample gently with small haemostat forceps or a hypodermic needle at the subcutaneous portion, lift from the surrounding tissue and cut free using sharp scissors.
- Place the sample in the correct transport medium. For normal histopathology, 10% neutral buffered formalin is used. For culture, consult the microbiology laboratory.
- Clean around biopsy sites with diluted 2% chlorhexidine or povidone-iodine (Betadine surgical scrub, SSL International) and suture using a single interrupted suture of 2–0 nylon. Clean and bandage the areas or apply antibiotic and protective topical creams or powders.

Other samples

Collection and examination and/or analysis of herbage and other materials available to the animals may also be valuable.

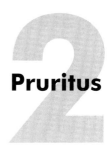

Pruritus

Pruritus is the commonest presenting sign in equine skin disease. It is manifested in many ways, which may be observed by the owner and deduced by the veterinary surgeon on examination of the affected animal(s). Such signs may include:

- Irritable demeanour.
- Restlessness.
- Kicking and stamping.
- Rubbing against objects.
- Biting the skin.
- Excoriation, exudation, crusting.
- Bruising, swelling, haematoma.
- Hair loss, thinning; broken hair.
- Skin thickening, scaling.

The severity of pruritus may be difficult to gauge from the history. Pruritus needs to be differentiated from pain. Some conditions combine both. Horses with painful lesions must be approached with great care. Sedation is sometimes necessary.

CONTAGIOUS CONDITIONS

Ectoparasitic infestation

Louse infestation

Clinical features
- Mild to severe pruritus, patchy alopecia, excoriation, exudation, in-contacts affected; ill temper, loss of condition and, if severe, anaemia (sucking lice only).

Werneckiella (Damalinia) equi
• Biting louse: small (c. 1.8 mm long) with a rounded head, many lice usually present; affects the dorso-lateral trunk and neck especially under the mane, and the head (Figure 2.1).

Haematopinus asini
• Sucking louse: large (c. 3.2 mm long), more visible, generally fewer lice; usually affects the base of the mane, tail, fetlocks. Populations can be high with very extensive infestations in long winter coats.

Diagnosis
• Signs, history (underlying problem causing debility?).
• Find lice and nits, and identify microscopically.

Treatment and control
• Topical insecticides containing cypermethrin (Deosan Deosect, Fort Dodge; Barricade, Sorex), permethrin (Fly Repellent Plus for Horses, Coopers, Schering-Plough Animal Health) and pyrethrins (Dermoline Shampoo for Horses, Day Son & Hewitt); pruritus stops in <36 h, transient urticaria has been reported.

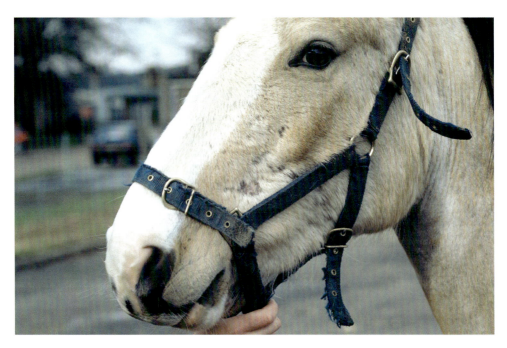

Figure 2.1 Alopecia, moth-eaten appearance, excoriations and hyper-pigmentation on horse with *Werneckiella* (*Damalinia*) infestation.

- *1% selenium sulphide shampoo (Seleen, CEVA Animal Health) shown to work for biting lice* (Paterson and Orrell, 1995). *Whole body shampooing repeated on three occasions at 10-day intervals with a contact time of 5–10 min before thorough rinsing.*
- *Ivermectin oral paste (e.g. Eqvalan, Merial; Furexel, Janssen; Panomec Paste for Horses, Merial), 200–300 µg/kg, repeated after 14 and 28 days for sucking lice* (Littlewood, 1999).
- Treat in-contacts, rugs, harness, saddlery.

Mite infestation

Chorioptic mange

Clinical features
- Infestation with *Chorioptes bovis* affects the distal parts of the limbs but may spread to other regions. The hind legs are more often involved and heavily feathered legs are especially susceptible.
- The problem is clinically apparent particularly during the colder times of the year.
- Affected animals show signs of pruritus with stamping, and rubbing or biting at the affected areas.
- Lesions (Figure 2.2) include scaling and crust formation in the pastern, fetlock and cannon regions.
- Exudative, proliferative dermatitis with secondary bacterial infection ('greasy heels') may develop in severe cases.

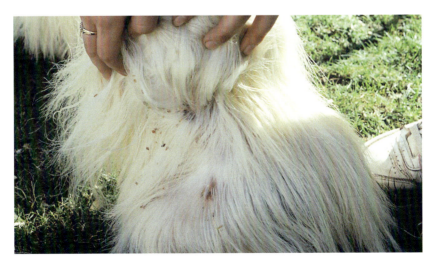

Figure 2.2 Haemorrhagic crusts and exudation affecting the pastern region of a Shire horse with chorioptic mange.

Diagnosis
- History and signs.
- Demonstrate the mite in scrapings from fresh lesions (Figure 2.3) which can often be found on the edges of more chronically affected skin.

Treatment (no licensed products)
Topical
- Clip the affected area first. The following treatments have been reported effective:
  - *1% selenium sulphide shampoo whole body washes (Seleen, CEVA Animal Health), repeated three times at 5-day intervals, allowing a skin contact time of 10 min prior to thorough rinsing* (Curtis, 1999).
  - *Fipronil (Frontline Spray; Merial Animal Health) applied so as to dampen the haircoat and skin surface* (Littlewood, 2000).
  - *6% Flumethrin (Bayticol Scab and Tick Dip, Bayer). Dilute 1:900 (66 µg/ml), apply up to 2 mg/kg (30 ml/kg), repeat after 14 days* (Littlewood, 1999).

Systemic
- *Ivermectin (Eqvalan Paste for Horses, Merial; Furexel, Janssen; Panomec Paste for Horses, Merial) at 200–300 µg/kg by mouth, may provide relief in 4–7 days and needs to be repeated after 10–14 days.* Treatment reduces the mite load by over 95% and provides an efficient means for the treatment of large groups of horses (Littlewood et al., 1995).
- Treat in-contacts and dispose of bedding to prevent reinfestation.

Sarcoptic and psoroptic mange

- May occur in imported horses; very rare in Western Europe.

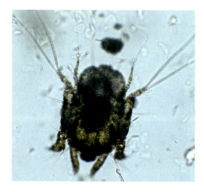

Figure 2.3 Adult female *Chorioptes bovis* in liquid paraffin (×125).

- *Sarcoptes scabiei* causes pruritus with papules, crusts, alopecia, excoriation and lichenification beginning on the head and neck and extending caudally.
- *Psoroptes equi* causes severe pruritus, crusting and alopecia, especially of the head (ears), mane and tail. Rapid transmission occurs.

Psoroptes cuniculi *infestation*

- Can be found in horses' ears and may cause no problems or lead to head shaking and ear rubbing. Affected animals may have a lop-eared appearance.

Diagnosis
- Signs and history indicate an ear problem. Mites can be obtained from deep within the ear and are visible as white moving dots. They can be identified by microscopy. Sedation and otoscopy may be necessary.

Treatment
- Clean debris and wax from ears. *Instil eardrops containing acaricide and repeat after 10 days.*

Free-living mites

Neotrombicula autumnalis *infestation*

Clinical features
- Larvae usually acquired from infested pasture in late summer or autumn.
- Can cause severe pruritus often indicated by stamping.
- Signs include papules, wheals and alopecia that may affect limbs, head and sometimes the ventral abdomen.
- Larvae may be visible as red dots (<0.5 mm) on affected skin (Figure 2.4).

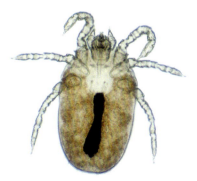

Figure 2.4 Larva of *Neotrombicula autumnalis* from a skin scraping.

Diagnosis
- History, signs, demonstration of the six-legged larvae in scrapings.

Treatment
- Larvae drop off after feeding but therapy is usually warranted. A single treatment with a topical antiparasitic preparation, e.g. *fipronil (Frontline Spray, Merial), cypermethrin (Deosan Deosect, Fort Dodge; Barricade, Sorex), permethrin (Fly Repellent Plus for Horses, Coopers, Schering-Plough Animal Health) or pyrethrins (Dermoline Shampoo for Horses, Day Son & Hewitt) is sufficient.*
- If possible, areas infested with these mites should be avoided in the late summer and autumn.

Forage mites

- These free-living mites, e.g. *Pyemotes* or *Acarus* spp., may be present in hay and bedding.
- Can cause papular and crusty lesions, which may be pruritic, in areas of skin in contact with the contaminated material (e.g. feet, muzzle).

Diagnosis
- Differentiate from other papular and crusting conditions affecting feet, muzzle.
- Demonstrate mites (0.3–0.6 mm long) in skin scrapings and samples of hay and bedding.

Treatment
- Replacement of contaminated material leads to recovery in a few days.

Dermanyssus gallinae *infestation*

- The red mite of poultry attacks at night and generally causes pruritus of the head and limbs. The mites are not normally present on the horse during the day.

Diagnosis
- Signs together with a history of contact with poultry housing are usually highly indicative.
- Mites are just visible with the naked eye. Examine scrapings and coat brushings taken at night.

Treatment
- As for *Neotrombicula autumnalis* infestation.
- Exclude contact with poultry. Horses may need to be moved away if the mite infestation cannot be eliminated.

Helminth infestation

Oxyuris equi

Clinical features
- Female worms emerge from the rectum and lay cream-coloured eggs on perineum causing pruritus.
- The horse rubs its tail (rat tail) and becomes restless or ill tempered.
- Infestation occurs especially in stabled horses where rapid transmission of the eggs can occur; eggs are sensitive to desiccation.

Diagnosis
- Signs are highly suggestive. Examine eggs using tape strip samples from the perianal region.
- Differentials: *Culicoides* hypersensitivity, other allergies, louse infestation.

Treatment and control
- Improve stable hygiene. A normal equine worming routine should give good control.
- Dealing with a specific infestation: ivermectin paste (Eqvalan Paste for Horses, Merial; Furexel, Janssen; Panomec Paste for Horses, Merial) given at 200–300 μg/kg by mouth twice at 3–6 week intervals, or moxidectin gel (Equest, Fort Dodge) at 0.4 mg/kg by mouth every 12 weeks.

Onchocercal dermatitis

Clinical features
- Now uncommon.
- Hypersensitivity (types I and III) to microfilariae affecting ventral midline, chest and withers.
- Pruritus, patchy alopecia, small papules, thickened dry scaly skin, poor hair regrowth, concentrated in ventral midline.
- If severe, marked pruritus, excoriation, crusts. Tail rubbing is rare.
- A summer problem.

Diagnosis
- History, signs.
- Biopsy and presence of helminth larvae (in skin with characteristic lesions).
- Examine minced skin, suspended in PBS for 3 h at 37°C, filter coarsely, centrifuge 5 min at 3000 rpm, examine deposit at 60–100× magnification for larvae.
- Differentials: sweet itch, trombiculidiasis. N.B. Insect hypersensitivity and onchocerciasis can both be associated with *Culicoides* and so may coexist.

Treatment

- Ivermectin paste (Eqvalan Paste for Horses; Merial, Furexel; Janssen, Panomec Paste for Horses; Merial) given at 200–300 μg/kg every 6–8 weeks or *moxidectin gel (Equest, Fort Dodge) 0.4 mg/kg every 12 weeks* (Monahan et al., 1995) is effective in killing the larvae. Most cases resolve with one treatment, however, regular treatment is needed as the adult worms are not killed and thus the condition may recur (Lyons et al., 1988; Scholl, 1998).
- Can give concurrent corticosteroids to lessen acute exacerbation that may be encountered within the first 3 days (Herd and Donham, 1988).

Larval nematode dermatitis

Clinical features

- Under unhygienic conditions (muddy yards, contaminated bedding) larvae of the free-living rhabditid nematode, *Pelodera strongyloides*, can invade equine skin and cause irritation.
- Marked pruritus, papules, pustules, ulcers, crusts, alopecia, erythema of limbs, ventrum.

Diagnosis

- Demonstrate motile nematode larvae in skin scrapings; biopsy specimens.

Treatment

- Clean and disinfect skin (e.g. can use antimicrobial cream). Signs regress over days to weeks. Clean and rectify environment.

Microbial infections

Microbial infections in which pruritus may be a feature are listed in Table 2.1. These conditions are considered in other sections of the book, as indicated.

Table 2.1 Microbial infections that may feature pruritus

Fungal disease	Causative organism	Bacterial disease	Causative organism
Superficial	Dermatophytes of the genera *Trichophyton* and *Microsporum*. *See Chapter 3*	Folliculitis and furunculosis	Pathogenic staphylococci; streptococci. *See Chapter 3*
		Botryomycosis	*See Chapter 5*
Deep	e.g. *Drechslera spicifera*, *Alternaria alternata*. *See Chapter 5*	Dermatophilosis	*Dermatophilus congolensis*. *See Chapter 3*

NON-CONTAGIOUS CONDITIONS

Insect attack in horses

Clinical features
- Insects involved: horse fly (*Tabanus*), stable fly (*Stomoxys*), midges (*Culicoides*), horn fly (*Haematobia*), black fly (*Simulium*), mosquitoes, wasps, bees.
- Signs may include:
  - Bite marks (Figure 2.5), bleeding, presence of a sting, pain, swelling.
  - Stamping, restlessness, irritability. Horses may choose to stand in smoke which drives away flies.

Treatment and control
- Depends on severity and pain.
- *Tabanus* and *Stomoxys*:
  - Topical anti-inflammatory or analgesic cream.
  - Sedation, e.g. acepromazine 0.08 mg/kg intramuscularly.
- Generally:
  - Repellents and/or persistent insecticides, e.g. synthetic pyrethroids.
  - Change environment – dispose of manure, cut vegetation, use environmental insecticides, depending on the life cycle of the insect(s) responsible, e.g. for *Tabanus* remove decaying vegetation and manure.

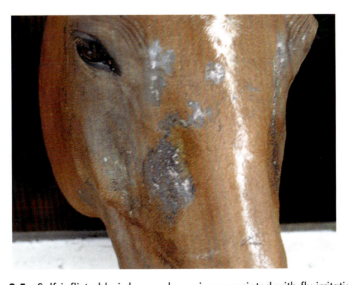

Figure 2.5 Self-inflicted hair loss and scarring associated with fly irritation.

Culicoides hypersensitivity

Synonyms: sweet itch, insect-bite hypersensitivity.

Clinical features

- Occurs in areas where *Culicoides* spp. attack occurs. Populations and attack are promoted by waterlogged ground and low wind speeds. Biting is diurnal and restricted to early morning and late afternoon in the summer and autumn in the UK.
- Hypersensitivity occurs principally in horses over 6 months of age.
- Signs include:
  - Pruritus indicated by rubbing and the presence of broken hairs especially in the mane and tail (Figures 2.6 and 2.7) (rat tail).
  - Papules, crusts, exudation and skin thickening dorsally (ears to tail); ventral lesions can occur (Figure 2.8). Note that some species of *Culicoides* bite ventral areas.
  - Horses may show irritability, restlessness and weight loss.

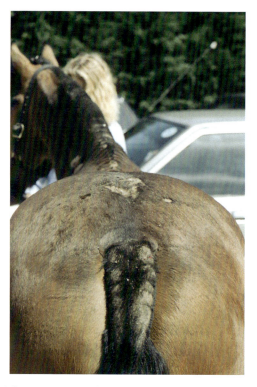

Figure 2.6   Hair loss, crusting and excoriation affecting the tail and sacral region in a horse with *Culicoides* hypersensitivity. Hair loss at the withers and of the mane can also be seen.

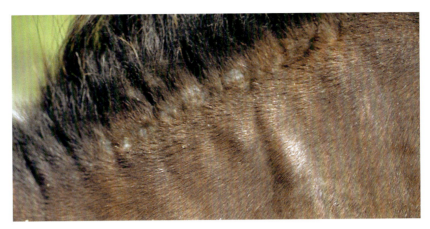

Figure 2.7 *Culicoides* hypersensitivity: alopecia of mane and body hairs, crusting and skin thickening.

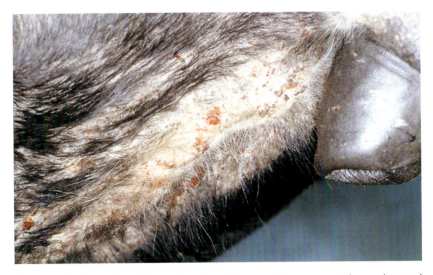

Figure 2.8 Ventral midline alopecia with excoriations, crusted papules and thickening in a pony with *Culicoides* hypersensitivity.

Diagnosis
- History, signs, presence of midges in the environment.
- Feeding midges burrow into mane and forelock to feed – part hair and search.
- Intradermal tests – cross-reaction occurs between different *Culicoides* spp. *Culicoides* extracts not readily available.
- Differentials: *Oxyuris equi* infestation, bites or hypersensitivity to other insects, atopy (may co-exist), contact dermatitis.

Management
- Prevent access to horses by *Culicoides*.
  - Stable horses between 4 p.m. and 8 a.m.
  - Cover horses with rugs and hoods.
  - Fine mesh screen for stables or install fans in stables to create a breeze.
  - Repellents and insecticides such as cypermethrin (Deosan Deosect, Fort Dodge: Barricade, Sorex), permethrin (Switch, Day Son & Hewitt; Fly Repellent Plus for Horses, Coopers, Schering-Plough Animal Health), residual insecticides, light oil, citronellol with permethrin or alone (Fly Repellent Plus for Horses, Coopers, Schering-Plough Animal Health; Extra Tail, Kalium).
  - Consider moving horses away from infested area.
- Anti-inflammatory and antipruritic therapy:
  - Antihistamines have limited effect. *Hydroxyzine hydrochloride (Atarax, Pfizer; 0.5–1 mg/kg by mouth, divided into three daily doses) is* said to be effective (Gortel, 1998).
  - Prednisolone or *methylprednisolone* at 1 mg/kg daily by mouth until control is achieved reducing to alternate day therapy if other measures do not adequately control the problem.
  - Topical soothing creams containing benzyl benzoate (Sweet itch lotion, Pettifer; Killitch, Carr & Day & Martin), shampoos containing *colloidal oatmeal (e.g. Episoothe, Virbac).*

Atopy

Clinical features
- Reactions to a wide variety of agents including pollens, moulds, dust and forage mites.
- Signs:
  - Recurrent pruritus and/or urticaria (Figure 2.9); variable seasonality. No other primary signs.
  - Secondary lesions: excoriation, scaling, alopecia, papules, lichenification, skin thickening, hyperpigmentation.

Diagnosis
- History, signs.
- Eliminate other pruritic diseases.
- Intradermal tests (Figure 2.10).
- Biopsy: superficial perivascular dermatitis, predominantly eosinophilic.
- Differentials: food hypersensitivity, ectoparasitic infestation, *Oxyuris* irritation, insect bite hypersensitivity, contact dermatitis.

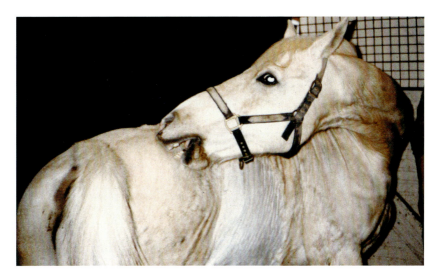

Figure 2.9   Intense pruritus in a horse with atopy, intradermal test positive to indoor (stable) allergens.

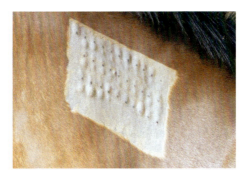

Figure 2.10   Intradermal test showing multiple positive reactions in an atopic horse.

Treatment and management

- Allergen avoidance, e.g. change bedding material, accommodation.
- Anti-inflammatory therapy:
  - Prednisolone at 1 mg/kg once daily by mouth until control achieved, then reduce to lowest dose alternate day regimen. Alternatively, *dexamethasone 0.02–0.1 mg/kg by mouth* (Opticorten, Novartis) *or intramuscularly as a loading dose with maintenance at 0.01–0.02 mg/kg every 48–72 h* (Rosenkrantz, 1998).
  - Antihistamines: not generally successful but *hydroxyzine hydrochloride (Atarax, Pfizer; 0.5–1 mg/kg by mouth, divided into three daily doses)* may be useful in chronic pruritus and urticaria.

- *Immunotherapy can be effective based on intradermal test results* (Rosenkrantz et al., 1998).
- Essential fatty acids do not seem useful generally but may help some horses.

Food allergy

Clinical features
- A poorly documented disease.
- May cause urticaria and pruritus.
- Diagnosis is rarely confirmed.

Diagnosis
- Exclude other pruritic and urticarial diseases.
- Carry out food exclusion trial for at least 3 weeks, e.g. only alfalfa hay.
- Confirm by provocative challenge.

Treatment and management
- Change diet.

Contact dermatitis

Clinical features
- Local lesions; allergic and irritant reactions may co-exist.
    - Pruritus.
    - Maculopapular rash, vesicles, exudation, crusting (Figure 2.11).

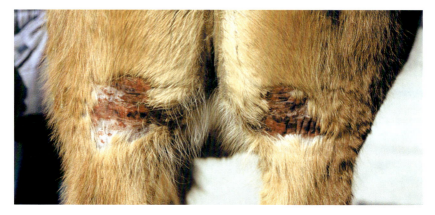

Figure 2.11   Irritant contact dermatitis caused by leaning against a fence coated with creosote.

- Contact sites affected. May relate to harness and tack. Promoted by moisture (sweating) and can affect both haired and hairless areas.
- Sensitisers include:
  - Dyes and preservatives, soaps, topical medicaments (insect repellents), plants and forage.

Diagnosis
- Signs, sites.
- Confirm by biopsy, patch tests, exclusion of suspected agent.

Management
- Remove source of allergen.
- Clean sites and apply topical glucocorticoids – short term.
- Systemic prednisolone at 1 mg/kg by mouth once daily until control achieved if allergen cannot be excluded.

Urticaria and angio-oedema

Clinical features
- Urticaria (Figure 2.12): wheals, varying in extent, which pit on pressure and are transient.
- Angio-oedema: large oedematous swellings involving leakage of serum or blood.
- Lesions especially on neck, trunk and head but can affect any part of the body. May be pruritic.

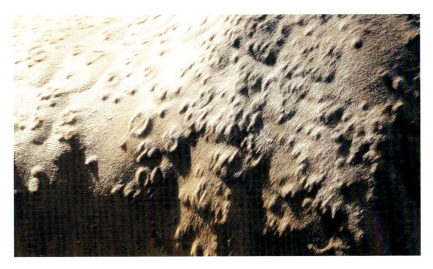

Figure 2.12   Urticaria. Multiple raised papules, plaques and annular lesions on the trunk and shoulder region.

- Causes: hypersensitivity, physical factors (light, heat, exercise, pressure), stress, topical and systemic drugs, chemicals (including soaps, leather conditioners) insect bites, infections (e.g. strangles, dermatophytosis), vaccines, feed.

Diagnosis
- History, signs, urticarial lesions pit on pressure, presence of causative factors, rule-outs. Biopsy not diagnostic but helps with rule-outs.

Management
- Eliminate cause:
  - Prednisolone at 1 mg/kg once daily until control achieved. Alternatively, *dexamethasone* (Opticorten, Novartis) *0.02–0.1 mg/kg as loading dose then maintained at 0.01–0.02 mg/kg every 48–72 h.*
- *Hydroxyzine hydrochloride (Atarax, Pfizer; 0.5–1 mg/kg by mouth, three times daily)* may be helpful.
- Prognosis:
  - Urticaria: good but often difficult to identify cause and may recur.
  - Angio-oedema: variable depending on severity and location.

Crusting and scaling

SEBORRHOEA

Crusts form when dried exudate, serum, purulent discharge, blood, cells or scales adhere to the skin surface. Scale is an accumulation of loose fragments of cornified cells. Normal loss of cornified cells is barely visible to the naked eye and the presence of scale indicates an abnormality of cornification. The presence of abnormal scaling is often termed **seborrhoea.**

Excessive scaling may be a feature of many skin diseases in the horse, including parasitic infestations, hypersensitivity diseases, and bacterial and fungal folliculitides. However, the predominant clinical sign in many of these conditions is pruritus, and these causes of secondary seborrhoea are covered elsewhere. Occult sarcoids, which may present with scaling as a major sign, are also covered elsewhere. Hepatic disease, malabsorption and nutritional deficiencies may also be accompanied by a secondary seborrhoea.

IDIOPATHIC SEBORRHOEA

There are several clinical syndromes where excessive scaling is the primary presenting sign, with no underlying disease evident. There is probably an underlying abnormality of cornification in these cases, which thus far has not been fully characterised.

Mane and tail seborrhoea

Clinical features
- An uncommon disorder characterised by moderate to severe scaling in the mane and/or tail regions.

- No age, breed or sex predilections reported.
- Scaling may be dry or oily and crust formation may be present.
- There is little or no accompanying pruritus but there may be some alopecia of the tail.
- Rule out the possibility of selenosis as a cause.

Treatment
- Treatment consists of frequent use of antiseborrhoeic shampoos. Examples are *Paxcutol (Virbac), Seleen (CEVA), Sebomild P (Virbac) and Coatex Medicated Shampoo (VetPlus)*.
- Initially there may be increased scaling followed by improvement.
- In some cases application of a humectant conditioner *(Humilac, Virbac)* may be beneficial as a rinse after, and between, bathing.

Generalised seborrhoea

- A rare skin disease; diagnosis can only be made when all causes of secondary seborrhoea have been ruled out. Treatment is as above.

Cannon keratosis

- Although also known as 'stud crud', there is no sex (or breed or age) predisposition, ruling out urine splatter as an aetiological factor.
- Signs:
  - Areas of scaling and crusting with variable alopecia, without pruritus or inflammation, affect the anterior aspect of both hind cannon bone regions. It is usually a lifelong affliction.

Treatment
- The condition is managed by regular application of topical antiseborrhoeic shampoos or lotions with antimicrobial activity *(Paxcutol, Sebomild P shampoo, Sebomild P lotion, Virbac; Seleen, Ceva; Coatex Medicated Shampoo, VetPlus)*.
- In severe cases topical glucocorticoids may be beneficial.

Linear keratosis and alopecia

Clinical features
- Quarter horses are predisposed to this characteristic skin condition, which is usually seen in young adult animals.

- Signs:
  - Lesions consist of asymptomatic, unilateral, vertical, linear band(s) of variably crusting and scaling alopecia predominantly affecting the neck and thorax. They may extend down the limbs.
- Histologically a lymphocytic mural folliculitis has been described.

Treatment
- Keratolytic shampoos or lotion and topical glucocorticoids may result in considerable temporary improvement. (Examples of shampoos and lotion: *Paxcutol, Sebomild P shampoo, Sebomild P lotion, Virbac; Seleen, Ceva; Coatex Medicated Shampoo, VetPlus*.)

INFECTIOUS CAUSES

Superficial fungal infection

Dermatophytosis

- Overdiagnosed. Diagnosis is often based on clinical signs, which can be deceptive. May occur sporadically or in outbreaks. Normally affects young horses.

Clinical features
Aetiology and specific features
- *Trichophyton equinum* var. *equinum* and *T. mentagrophytes* commonly responsible.
  - Incubation period usually about 10 days but may be up to 4 weeks.
  - **Can be very pruritic** especially in 'girth itch'. A scratch reflex can often be elicited.
  - Spontaneous recovery generally occurs in 5–6 weeks but lesions may be prolonged if secondary infection is present. Course is generally longer in horses under 4 years old.
- *Microsporum equinum*.
  - Causes a milder syndrome than *T. equinum* and *T. mentagrophytes*.
  - Sometimes wrongly identified as *M. canis*.
- *Microsporum gypseum*.
  - Usually less severe, less pruritic and more focal than the other dermatophytes, but may be more widespread.
  - Can be transmitted by tabanid flies.
- Other dermatophytes occasionally cause disease.
- Signs:
  - May show lesions resembling urticaria initially. Tends to be localised and focal or multifocal. Erythema may be visible in

non-pigmented skin. Hairs are typically raised; lesions extend centrifugally. Scaling, crusting and hair loss develop (Figures 3.1 and 3.2). Crusts may be quite thick (5 mm) and can be grossly indistinguishable from those of dermatophilosis, however *Dermatophilus* does not damage the hairs. On recovery hair regrowth usually starts at the centre of lesions.

– Lesions are pruritic to non-pruritic.

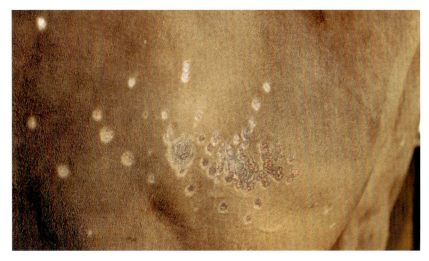

Figure 3.1   *Trichophyton* infection. Multiple annular lesions of alopecia, scaling and crusting.

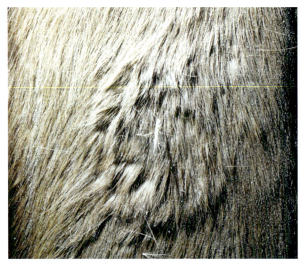

Figure 3.2   Crusted lesions with hair tufts in a case of *Trichophyton equinum* infection. (Courtesy of *Veterinary Record*.)

Diagnosis

- History, especially evidence of transmission to and/or from other animals or humans.
- Signs.
- Confirmation:
  - Examine crusts and hairs. Rule out dermatophilosis (impression smears). Demonstrate arthroconidia and/or hyphae.
  - Collect crusts and hairs for dermatophyte culture and species identification. Note that *T. equinum* var. *equinum* has a specific requirement for niacin, which may need to be added to the culture medium.
  - Hairs infected with *M. equinum* exhibit yellow-green fluorescence under the Wood's lamp.
- Differentials: dermatophilosis, staphylococcal folliculitis, pemphigus foliaceus.

Treatment and management

- Spontaneous recovery makes assessment of the efficacy of therapy difficult.
- As the disease is zoonotic, topical therapy is advisable to kill exposed organisms and to reduce spread to other animals and contamination of the environment.
- Efficacy of therapy should be checked by clinical examination (disappearance of lesions) and then by sampling (Mackenzie brush technique useful) and culture.
- Spores can survive for months on hair shafts and in crusts.

Topical therapy

- Enilconazole (Imaverol, Janssen). Wash with a 0.2% solution every 3 days on four occasions.
- Natamycin (Mycophyt, Intervet). Spray (1 litre per adult animal) or local application using a 0.01% solution, repeat after 4–5 days and again in 14 days if necessary. Treated animals should not be exposed to sunlight for several hours. Avoid metal containers as natamycin reacts with heavy metals.
- *Miconazole and chlorhexidine shampoo (Malaseb, Leo)* (Paterson, 1997). *Affected horses are shampooed twice weekly and animals in contact once weekly*. Expect resolution within 5 weeks.
- Note that topical therapy is unlikely to kill all arthrospores within hair follicles necessitating repeated treatment as infected hairs grow.
- Systemic therapy – registered products include:
  - Griseofulvin, 10 mg/kg of oral powder, granules or paste; *duration of 7 days may be quoted but 3–12 weeks needed*. Contra-indications: renal and hepatic impairment, pregnancy. Use gloves. Should not be handled by women of childbearing age.

Control of dermatophytosis
- Hygiene:
  - Disinfect accommodation, boxes, tack. Look for and eliminate source of infection, including infected humans.
  - Environmental treatment with imidazole foggers [Fungaflor (imazalil), Hortichem] and potassium monopersulphate sprays (Virkon, Antec International) can be used to reduce contamination.
- Isolation and quarantine:
  - Prevent transmission to other animals, people.

Prophylaxis
- Live vaccines against *Trichophyton* spp. have been used with success in other species and may become available for the horse.

BACTERIAL INFECTION

Folliculitis and furunculosis

Associated with bacterial infection involving pathogenic staphylococci and streptococci.

- *S. intermedius, S. aureus, S. hyicus.*
- *Streptococcus equi, Strep. equisimilis, Strep. zooepidemicus.*

Clinical features
- Papules which may develop into pustules, oedema, exudation and crusting, particularly in warm weather and affecting the saddle region and areas in contact with tack (Figures 3.3 and 3.4).

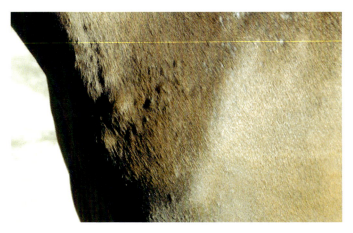

Figure 3.3   Staphylococcal folliculitis and furunculosis.

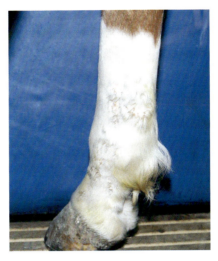

Figure 3.4   Bacterial folliculitis of pastern and metatarsal regions. Staphylococci and streptococci were isolated.

- Lesions may coalesce and sometimes form abscesses if complicated, e.g. foreign body reactions, cheek abscesses.
- Usually associated with rubbing or pressure from ill-fitting harness and saddle cloths, and heavy work; poor hygiene may be a factor.
- Usually painful, sometimes pruritic.
- Localised syndromes.
  - Pastern folliculitis affecting the caudal aspect of the pastern and fetlock of one or more limbs. Differentiate from other causes of 'greasy heels'.
  - Tail pyoderma affects the dorsal region and is often associated with pruritus and rubbing. Difficult to treat.
  - Limb cellulitis is sometimes seen in race horses.

Diagnosis
- Biopsy; isolation of bacteria from biopsy specimens or deep within the lesion is recommended.
- Differentials: dermatophytosis, dermatophilosis.

Management and therapy
- Rest from work.
- Wash skin daily with antiseptics for about 7 days and then every 3–4 days until resolution.
  - Povidone iodine or chlorhexidine. *Chlorhexidine scrub (Hibiscrub Veterinary, Schering-Plough) can be used diluted about 1 in 4. Lather and cleanse the lesions, allow 10 min contact and then rinse thoroughly.* Other

antimicrobial agents that may be used include *chlorhexidine and miconazole (Malaseb, Leo), chloroxylenol (Coatex Medicated Shampoo, VetPlus), ethyl lactate (Etiderm, Virbac), piroctone olamine (Sebomild P, Virbac).*

- Systemic antibiotics, e.g.:
  - *Trimethoprim and sulphadiazine paste (Equitrim Equine Paste, Boehringer Ingelheim; Tribrissen Oral Paste, Schering-Plough), 15 mg/kg twice daily for 2 weeks.*
  - *Procaine penicillin, 15–20 mg/kg twice daily by intramuscular injection for 10 days.*
  - Ceftiofur (Excenel, Pfizer Animal Health), 2 mg/kg once daily.
  - Oral enrofloxacin can be used for longer-term therapy (but not in immature horses). *Baytril 10% Oral Solution (Bayer) is used at 5.0–7.5 mg/kg once daily.* This is a poultry preparation not licensed for the horse.
- Disinfect tack thoroughly.
- Correct any management problems. Look for and eliminate sources of infection.

Dermatophilosis

Clinical features
- Clinical syndromes:
  - Rain scald – affects dorsal trunk.
  - Mud fever or rash, greasy heels – affect pasterns and other parts of the distal limbs (Figure 3.5).

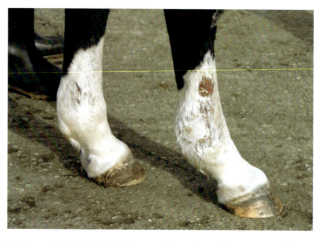

Figure 3.5 Dermatophilosis. Erythema, alopecia and crusting in the white-haired lateral surface of the limb.

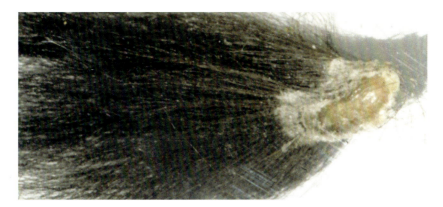

Figure 3.6 Thick scab with attached hair from a lesion of dermatophilosis.

- – Lesions of the face and muzzle, perineum also occur.
- Generally occurs in warm, wet weather, especially autumn and winter and following prolonged and/or heavy rain.
- Any trauma to the skin will predispose to infection, e.g. grooming, gravel thrown up by hooves, sharp vegetation. Non-pigmented skin is predisposed.
- Recurs in previously affected horses and spreads to in-contacts.
- Lesion development.
  - – Focal paintbrush lesions develop into thick crusts (Figures 3.6 and 3.7), with a concave undersurface covered by a thin layer of pus.
  - – Long coats may disguise the extent of the lesions.
  - – Hairs are not damaged but are epilated leading to alopecia when crusts are removed. Regrowth is not affected.
  - – In wet areas the crusts may not remain attached. Prolonged wetting of the skin leading to maceration may allow secondary infection. When this involves the limbs it may result in oedema and cellulitis.

Diagnosis
- History, signs, impression smears (Gram's or Giemsa stain). The appearance of *Dermatophilus* is diagnostic (Gram-positive, branching filaments, breaking up into multiple rows of cocci; Figure 3.8). The vigorously motile zoospores may be visible in crushed scabs emulsified in water.
- Material from the crusts can be cultured but it is difficult to isolate the slow-growing *Dermatophilus*.
- Differentials: other causes of greasy heels, dermatophytosis, pastern folliculitis, photosensitisation, contact dermatitis, pastern leucocytoclastic vasculitis.

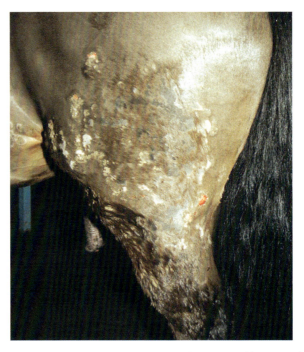

Figure 3.7 Dermatophilosis. Raised crusts and matting of hair, patchy alopecia and areas of ulceration with haemorrhagic and purulent exudation.

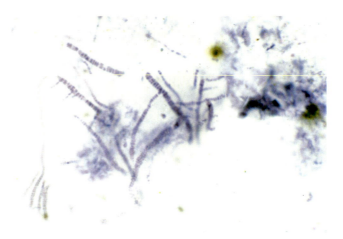

Figure 3.8 Giemsa-stained smear from an emulsified scab. Note the characteristic branching filaments composed of parallel rows of cocci.

Therapy and management
- Bring in to dry housing.
- Rectify or treat underlying problems.
- Remove crusts with keratolytic shampoos or manually; hairs remain attached to the crusts and may need to be cut to aid detachment. Sedation may be necessary.
- Dispose of crusts properly, as they are a new source of infection.
- Use twice daily washes with topical antibacterials, e.g. *chlorhexidine scrub diluted to 1–2%, lathered, left for 10 min and then rinsed thoroughly or chlorhexidine and miconazole shampoo (Malaseb, Leo)*, followed by drying.
- Systemic antibiotic (5 days at the standard dose) may be needed if severe or when other infections are involved. Systemic treatment allows healing at the skin surface and separation of the crusts over a period of days; they can then be more easily removed.
- Lesions on the distal parts of the limbs can be very painful. Pain and inflammation may be relieved by the use of topical glucocorticoid creams.
- Warn owners and plan for recurrence in future periods of wet weather.
- Isolate affected animals and disinfect tack to avoid spread to other animals and humans. Most disinfectants will readily kill *Dermatophilus*.

VIRAL INFECTION

Aural plaques

See Chapter 4.

IMMUNE-MEDIATED CAUSES

Pemphigus foliaceus

Clinical features
- Antibodies directed against epidermal cell surface antigens result in loss of intercellular cohesion and the formation of intraepidermal vesicles or vesicopustules.
- This is a relatively common immune-mediated skin disease in the horse. The Appaloosa breed may be predisposed.
- There is no sex predisposition.
- Age of onset is important with respect to the prognosis. Cases in animals less than one year of age tend to be less severe, respond well to therapy and may spontaneously regress.

- Signs:
  - Whilst the primary lesion is a vesicle or vesicopustule, the usual presentation is of a crusting, scaling dermatosis that often begins on the face and limbs, but commonly becomes generalised (Figures 3.9 and 3.10).

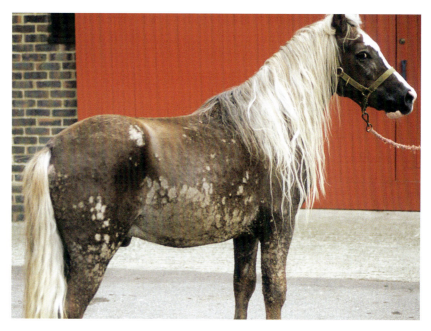

Figure 3.9 Generalised crusting and alopecia in a stallion with pemphigus foliaceus.

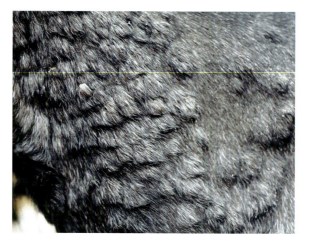

Figure 3.10 Crusting and matted tufts of hair in a young pony with widespread pemphigus foliaceus.

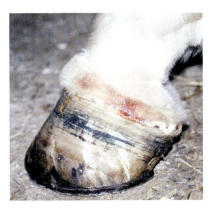

Figure 3.11 Crusting and haemorrhagic erosion and ulceration affecting the coronary band of a 14-year-old horse with pemphigus foliaceus.

- In some cases lesions are limited to the coronary band, chestnut and ergot regions (Figure 3.11). Intact vesicles are difficult to find. Lesions consist of areas of focal crusting, annular erosions and alopecia.
- Oedema of the extremities and ventrum may be present, often out of proportion to the surface skin changes. Although mucocutaneous sites are often involved the mucosal surfaces are rarely affected.
- Concurrent systemic signs of fever, depression and anorexia are seen in severe cases. Variable pruritus or pain may be present.

Diagnosis
- Cytological examination of vesicle or pustule contents reveals the presence of acantholytic keratinocytes and non-degenerate neutrophils and/or eosinophils with an absence of bacteria.
- Diagnostic investigations should include microscopical examination of hair and crusts, bacterial and fungal culture, and multiple skin biopsies for histopathology.
- Histologically the primary lesion is an intraepidermal or subcorneal vesicopustule containing acantholytic cells together with neutrophils, although sometimes eosinophils may predominate.
- Since these lesions are fragile they are transient and the only clue to the diagnosis may be the presence of large numbers of acantholytic keratinocytes in the surface crusts.
- Autoantibodies can be demonstrated by direct immunofluorescence or immunohistochemical techniques in 50–75% of cases, which have not received corticosteroids.
- Differentials: dermatophilosis, dermatophytosis, systemic granulomatous disease and idiopathic seborrhoea.

Treatment
- The disease in young horses carries a good prognosis and treatment usually secures lifelong remission.
- In the older horse, even though the initial response to treatment may be good, permanent maintenance therapy is required.
  - Owing to the need for lifelong therapy and the nature and expense of the drugs involved, it is essential that owners are aware of the implications at the outset.
- Corticosteroids are the treatment of choice.
  - Either prednisolone at a dose of 1–2 mg/kg daily by mouth or *dexamethasone (Opticorten, Novartis) 0.2 mg/kg per day by mouth or by injection dropping to 0.1 mg/kg after 24 h.*
  - Once lesions are improving (no new lesions) the dose of steroids can be gradually reduced, by about 20% per week.
  - Too rapid reduction allows recurrence of lesions, which may be resistant to subsequent treatment.
  - Once the minimum daily dose required to keep the disease in remission is reached *alternate day prednisolone, beginning at double the effective daily dose, should be used for maintenance.*
- Gold therapy:
  - If the condition is resistant to corticosteroids or the maintenance dose required is unacceptably high, *chrysotherapy (gold salts), e.g. sodium aurothiomalate (Myocrisin, JHC), can be given by deep intramuscular injection at a dose rate of 1 mg/kg once weekly, after two test doses of 20 and 40 mg one week apart.*
  - There is a lag phase of several weeks before a response is seen.
  - Once in remission the frequency of injections may be reduced. Side effects including blood dyscrasias, proteinuria and skin eruptions are described in other species, and monitoring of the haemogram and urinalysis is advised.
  - *Azathioprine has been used successfully* but is expensive.

Cutaneous lupus erythematosus

Clinical features
- Classically lupus erythematosus is divided into two forms, chronic cutaneous (discoid) lupus erythematosus (DLE) involving the skin and occasionally mucous membranes, and systemic lupus erythematosus (SLE), which is a multisystemic disease with frequent skin involvement.
- DLE may represent a benign variant of SLE.

- The cutaneous signs and dermatohistopathology of DLE and SLE in the horse are similar and thus the disease may be best referred to as cutaneous lupus erythematosus (CLE).
- Relatively rare. Various factors including genetic predisposition, hormones, ultraviolet light, immune dysfunction and viral infections may be involved in the aetiology.
- Usually occurs in adult horses with no known breed or sex predilection.
- Signs:
  - Major sign is depigmentation, with patchy alopecia and varying degrees of erythema and scaling.
  - Lesions commonly found on the face, around the eyes, lips and nostrils; perineal and genital areas may also be involved. In long-standing cases the skin may appear like 'wrinkled parchment'.
  - The alopecia of haired areas is usually cicatricial (scarring) and permanent. Sunlight may exacerbate lesions.
  - Systemic involvement is rare but fever, weight loss, proteinuria, haemolytic anaemia, thrombocytopenia and arthropathy may be encountered.

Diagnosis
- Histopathological examination and immunofluorescence or immuno-histochemistry of biopsies of affected skin.
  - Histopathological changes are centred on the dermo-epidermal junction and can be difficult to interpret.
  - Immunoglobulin (IgM and/or IgG) and complement (C3) may be demonstrated in a linear band at the basement membrane.
- In most cases a positive antinuclear antibody (ANA) titre is reported. Routine haematology, a biochemical panel and urinalysis should be performed to detect other organ involvement.
- Differentials:
  - CLE must be considered in any disease where depigmentation involves mucocutaneous junctions.
  - A major differential would be idiopathic leukoderma (vitiligo) of mature Arab horses and the presence of any inflammatory signs (erythema, scaling) in such a horse would strongly indicate the possibility of CLE.

Treatment
- CLE without systemic involvement can be managed by avoidance of sunlight (stabling, use of topical sunscreens) and by the use of topical corticosteroids (e.g. *1% hydrocortisone*).

- Cases with systemic involvement have been treated with prednisolone at initial doses of 1 mg/kg twice daily by mouth, reducing to the lowest possible dose on an alternate day basis. However, response to therapy is unpredictable and the prognosis guarded.

Hyperaesthetic leukotrichia

See also Chapter 7.

Clinical features
- Also known as 'dorsal midline erythema multiforme'.
- This is an uncommon but characteristic skin disease with no age, breed or sex predisposition. In some cases there is an association with the use of rhinopneumonitis vaccine.
- Signs:
  - Lesions may be single or multiple and are found on the midline between the withers and tail base.
  - They consist of focal crusts approximately 1–5 mm in diameter.
  - There is a marked degree of pain associated with this condition, which may precede the development of crusts.
  - Within a few weeks white hairs appear at the site of lesions, the pain subsides; crusts disappear over a period of 1–3 months. The leukotrichia is permanent.

Diagnosis
- The clinical appearance is usually distinctive. Confirm with histopathology.

Treatment
- Corticosteroids, even at high doses, are of only limited value. The disease usually runs its own course.

Drug eruption

See Chapter 4.

ENVIRONMENTAL CAUSES

Irritant contact dermatitis

Clinical features
- Contact dermatitis due to non-allergic causes may occur as a result of mechanical abrasion of the skin due to ill-fitting or

poorly maintained tack or working the horse in a muddy or gritty terrain.
- Chemical contact dermatitis most commonly follows the inappropriate application of skin medicaments, exposure to stable disinfectants, or in association with cleaning agents used on harness or stable blankets.
- Occasionally accidental exposure to caustic or corrosive chemicals may be encountered.
- Signs:
  - Severity is dependent upon the nature of the irritant involved, but a low-grade inflammation accompanied by scaling, hair loss and variable irritation is common.
  - More severe reactions present with blistering, hair loss, oedema, exfoliation and weeping erosions or ulcerations.
  - Lesions are confined to the contact areas and, together with the history, usually give an indication as to the nature of the causative agent.

Treatment
- Further exposure to the agent must be prevented.
- It may be necessary to remove the agent from the skin surface by washing.
- Symptomatic palliative therapy may be required (anti-inflammatory drugs, protective dressings, control of secondary infection).

Toxicoses

- Crusting and scaling of the skin are common signs in several chemical toxicoses. Hair loss is also commonly seen, and may be more prominent than the scaling – *see* Chapter 6 (arsenic, mercury and selenium toxicoses).

Iodism

Clinical features
- Iodine toxicosis usually follows excessive administration of iodides in the treatment of cutaneous mycoses.
- Signs are generalised dryness and scaling of the skin with variable alopecia, and watering of the eyes and nose.
- Iodine is rapidly metabolised and excreted, and once the source of iodine is removed the condition resolves.

UNCERTAIN AETIOLOGY

Generalised (systemic) granulomatous disease [equine sarcoidosis (not to be confused with equine sarcoids)]

Clinical features
- Characterised by generalised granuloma formation and appears analogous to human sarcoidosis.
- Aetiology: unknown but presumed to be an abnormal host response to some unidentified antigen(s). The role of the plant, hairy vetch, is uncertain.
- Signs:
  - Skin involvement in most cases.
  - Cutaneous lesions most commonly consist of scaling and crusting with variable alopecia, which may be focal, multifocal or generalised (Figures 3.12 and 3.13).
  - Nodular lesions are less common but may co-exist with the scaling lesions.
- Systemic signs:
  - Weight loss, decreased appetite and a persistent, low-grade fever are common.
  - Internal organ involvement may include the lungs, lymph nodes, liver, gastrointestinal tract, spleen, kidney, bones and central nervous system (CNS).

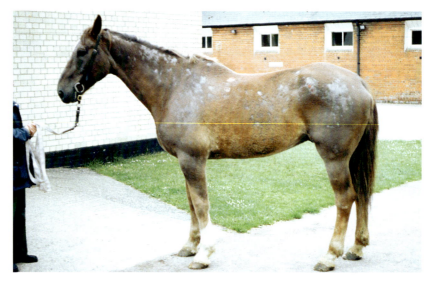

Figure 3.12   Generalised patchy alopecia and scaling in a 9-year-old with generalised granulomatous disease. Note poor bodily condition. Lymphadenopathy was also present.

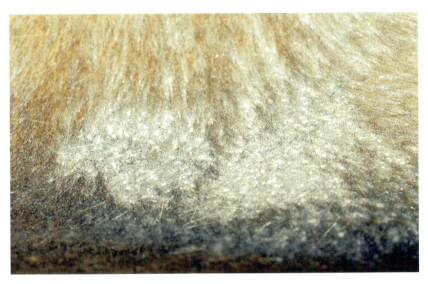

Figure 3.13   Cutaneous lesions in generalised granulomatous disease.

Diagnosis
- Laboratory findings:
  - May include leucocytosis, mild anaemia, elevated fibrinogen, hyperglobulinaemia, and abnormal hepatic and renal function.
- Histopathology:
  - Diagnosis confirmed by identification of typical non-caseating granulomas comprised of epithelioid and giant cells. These are found in all organs involved.
  - Biopsies of skin and peripheral lymph node are of greatest value.
  - No aetiological agent is found on special staining.

Treatment
- Little has been published on the management of this condition, but corticosteroids are probably the treatment of choice, at immuno-suppressive doses (e.g. prednisolone, 1–2 mg/kg once daily reducing to the same dose or less every other day).
- The disease appears to be more severe in the horse than in man, where two thirds of cases undergo spontaneous regression.

Exfoliative eosinophilic dermatitis and stomatitis or enteritis

Clinical features
- Characterised by tissue eosinophilia affecting the skin, oral cavity, salivary glands, pancreas, gastrointestinal tract, bronchial and biliary epithelium. The aetiology is unknown.

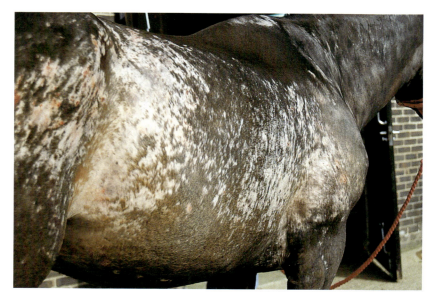

Figure 3.14   Sealing, crusting, excoriation and alopecia on the trunk of a horse with exfoliative eosinophilic dermatitis and stomatitis.

- Signs:
  - Skin lesions characterised by exudation, scaling and crusting with alopecia (Figure 3.14).
  - Coronary band, face and oral mucosa are affected initially with progression to a generalised exfoliative dermatitis.
  - Intense pruritus with self-mutilation present in some horses.
  - Chronic weight loss is common, often without loss of appetite. Loose faeces may be passed. Dependent oedema may be present.
  - Affected horses are usually dull and lethargic, and may be febrile.
  - Thickened bowel wall, thickened mesentery and enlarged lymph nodes may be detected on rectal examination.

Diagnosis
- Biopsies of skin show eosinophilic infiltration of a non-specific nature. Rectal mucosal biopsies may show similar infiltration.
- Low total plasma protein and albumin concentrations, reduced carbohydrate absorption.
- Differentials: pemphigus foliaceus, bullous pemphigoid, SLE, generalised granulomatous disease (equine sarcoidosis), vasculitis, dermatophilosis, dermatophytosis.

Treatment
• Glucocorticoids may provide some temporary relief. No known effective therapy and recovery not recorded.

'Greasy heels' syndrome

Clinical features
• A variety of inflammatory skin conditions may affect the lower limb and pastern region of the horse, and a number of terms may be used to describe the syndrome including grease or greasy heels, cracked heels, scratches and mud fever.
• None of these terms refers to a specific disease entity. They describe a clinical presentation that is common to a number of diseases.
• Signs:
  – Non-pigmented extremities are often involved or more severely involved.
  – Initial lesions affect the palmar or plantar aspect of the pastern region but may extend to the dorsal aspect of the limb and proximally.
  – Erythema, oozing and hair loss are common early signs progressing to crust formation (Figure 3.15).
  – Ulceration may occur with underlying vasculitis.
  – Chronically, thickening of the skin and fissure formation develops.

Diagnosis
• It is essential that a definitive diagnosis be reached so that proper therapeutic measures can be instigated.
• A full medical history should be taken.

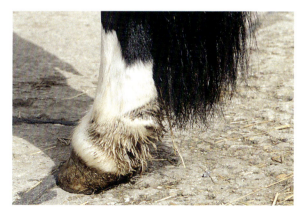

Figure 3.15 Exudative pastern dermatitis – 'greasy heels'.

- Liver enzymes and bile acids should be evaluated if lesions are restricted to non-pigmented skin.
- Crusts and scrapes should be examined for *Dermatophilus* organisms, fungal elements and *Chorioptes* mites, and submitted for bacterial and fungal culture.
- Skin biopsies may be indicated, for conventional histopathology and immunofluorescence or immunohistochemistry.
- Biopsy samples should also be submitted for bacterial and fungal culture. Beware of damaging the tendon sheaths that are superficial in the palmar or plantar pastern regions.
- Differentials: irritant contact dermatitis or hypersensitivity, pastern folliculitis, dermatophilosis, dermatophytosis, chorioptic mange, trombiculidiasis, horsepox, photosensitivity, vasculitis, exfoliative eosinophilic dermatitis and enteritis or stomatitis, idiopathic pastern dermatitis.

Treatment
- Depends upon the cause but should include:
  - Removal of crusts (*see* section on dermatophilosis) and thorough cleansing, prevention of further damage by irritants, moisture and sunlight. Astringent or caustic compounds should be avoided.
  - Topical anti-inflammatory preparations with antibacterial and antifungal activities are frequently used. *2% chlorhexidine and 2% miconazole shampoo (Malaseb, Leo), diluted at ratio of 1:2 and applied twice daily*, can be used as a topical antibacterial and antifungal rinse. Ensure adequate contact time and thoroughly dry area after rinsing.
  - Stable horse on clean, dry, soft bedding.
  - If vasculitis is identified aggressive systemic corticosteroid therapy is indicated.
- In idiopathic cases, cleansing and protection of affected areas with judicious use of corticosteroids may be the best approach.

Ulcers and erosions

CONTAGIOUS CAUSES

Helminth infestation

Cutaneous habronemiasis (summer sores)

Clinical features
- Seen more in temperate and tropical climates.
- Rarely recognised in the UK.
- Transmitted by insects.
- Seasonal incidence of warmer months.

Cause:
- *Habronema muscae, H. microstoma, H. megastoma*.
  - Adult worms live in equine stomach. Larvae passed in faeces and ingested by flies acting as intermediate hosts (*Musca domestica*, the housefly, and *Stomoxys calcitrans*, the stable fly). Flies deposit infective larvae around horse's lips and they are swallowed to complete normal life cycle.
  - Cutaneous disease results from aberrant parasitism when larvae are deposited in damaged skin or possibly mucous membranes.
  - Hypersensitivity response believed to be involved.

Signs:
- Ulcerative or proliferative lesions around eyes, distal extremities and external genitalia.
- Individual horses affected.

Diagnosis
- Diagnostic indicators:
  - History, clinical signs and seasonal occurrence.

- Confirmatory tests:
  - Skin biopsy to show larvae or characteristic eosinophilic response within tissue.
  - Microscopy of sediment from superficial scrapings or washings suspended in normal saline, following centrifugation.
- Differential diagnoses:
  - Exuberant granulation tissue, squamous cell carcinoma, fibroblastic sarcoid, infectious granulomata.

Treatment and management
Therapeutic approach
- Ivermectin (Eqvalan Paste for Horses, Merial; Furexel, Janssen; Panomec Paste; Merial) at 200 µg/kg by mouth given twice at 3–6 week intervals kills most larvae and produces rapid resolution of lesions. Prophylaxis depends on fly control. Steroids are also effective when used in conjunction with ivermectin.
- In cases with excessive exuberant granulation it may be necessary to surgically remove the tissue and bandage (if necessary), with judicious use of antibiotics and topical steroids.
- Prognosis:
  - Good.
- Prophylaxis:
  - Insect control.
  - Regular deworming.

Viral infections

Coital exanthema

Clinical features
- Caused by equine herpes virus (EHV)-3, the disease is spread by coitus, fomites and insect vectors.
- Signs:
  - Lesions consist of papules and vesicles, which may ulcerate and crust, affecting the penis, prepuce and scrotum of males (Figure 4.1), and the vulva and perineum of females.
  - Lips, mouth and nostrils may also be involved.
  - Healing is usually complete in 14 days, although focal depigmentation (*see* Chapter 7) may persist. Secondary bacterial infection may complicate the primary lesions.
  - Lesions may recur.

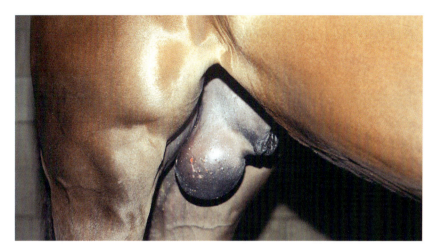

Figure 4.1   Coital exanthema showing epidermal vesicles and marked scrotal swelling.

Diagnosis
- Coital exanthema must be differentiated from other viral infections and immune-mediated conditions such as bullous pemphigoid, and other genital infections.
- Biopsy specimens reveal ballooning degeneration of basal epithelium and vesicle formation. Intranuclear inclusion bodies may be identified.
- Definitive diagnosis can be confirmed by virus isolation from vesicle contents, crusts or biopsy samples, identification of virus in samples by electron microscopy, or demonstration of a rising antibody titre to EHV-3.

Treatment
- Stud animals should be rested from coitus for a minimum of 4 weeks.
- Secondary infection should be treated if present.
- Topical antiseptic bathing and emollient creams may be beneficial.

Horse pox

Clinical features
- A rare, benign disease of horses in Europe. The aetiological agent is an unclassified poxvirus antigenically related to cowpox virus.
- Signs: three clinical presentations are described.
  - Oral lesions.
  - Pastern and fetlock lesions.
  - Vulvar lesions.

- Lesions consist of vesicles, umbilicated pustules and crusts affecting the skin and mucosal surfaces.
- Mild pyrexia may occur.
- Horses with limb involvement may be lame.

Diagnosis
- Ballooning degeneration of epidermal cells is seen on biopsy, with intraepidermal vesicles and intracytoplasmic inclusion bodies.
- Demonstration of poxvirus by electron microscopy and virus isolation confirm the diagnosis.

Treatment
- The natural course of the disease is 2–4 weeks and recovered horses have long-term immunity.

Immune-mediated causes

Bullous pemphigoid

Clinical features
- A rare auto-immune disease of horses resulting from auto-antibodies directed against antigens at the dermo-epidermal junction.
- Signs:
  - The primary lesions are vesicles or bullae that rapidly ulcerate, affecting skin, mucocutaneous junctions and oral mucosa. The axillary and inguinal areas are particularly affected.
  - Ulcers, crusts and epidermal collarettes are the usual signs, with variable pruritus or pain.
  - There may be anorexia, fever and depression, and excessive salivation if oral involvement is significant.

Diagnosis
- Biopsy findings of subepidermal vesicular dermatitis are strongly suggestive.
- Direct immunofluorescence or immunohistochemistry may demonstrate linear deposits of immunoglobulin and, usually, complement at the dermo-epidermal junction, in the absence of previous steroid therapy.
- Differentials include: viral diseases such as horse pox, herpes coital exanthema and vesicular stomatitis, cutaneous lupus erythematosus, erythema multiforme and drug eruptions.

Treatment
- The prognosis is grave with poor response to immunosuppressive doses of corticosteroids.

Erythema multiforme

- Recently recognised in the horse and at present considered an infrequently occurring dermatosis.
- Erythema multiforme (EM) occurs secondary to a number of preceding factors or diseases the most common of which are:
  - Drugs (including non-medicinal chemicals).
  - Infections (viral, esp. herpes, fungal and bacterial).
  - Malignancy.
- The pathogenesis is very similar to that of the graft-versus-host reaction.
- Signs:
  - EM is an acute and sometimes recurrent dermatosis, ranging in severity from mild to severe.
  - Lesions tend to be symmetrically distributed and mucous membranes may be involved.
  - Whilst the clinical appearance can be wide ranging, the basic lesion is either macular or vesicular.
  - Since vesicles are short-lived, lesions are usually focal or multifocal erosions and ulcerations or crusts at presentation.

Diagnosis

- A careful history is essential, noting previous drug administration and previous or concurrent illnesses.
- Histopathology:
  - Reveals necrotic (apoptotic) keratinocytes in the epidermis and adnexal epithelium; lymphocytic exocytosis and satellitosis; vacuolar change of the basal cell layer and/or basement membrane zone; oedema of the superficial dermis; extravasated erythrocytes in the superficial dermis; superficial perivascular lymphohistiocytic infiltrate.
  - Subepidermal vesicle formation may arise due to vacuolar degeneration and/or severe superficial dermal oedema.
  - The apoptosis of keratinocytes may be very extensive.
- Differentials: all diseases showing erosions or ulcers of the oral mucosa, mucocutaneous junctions, cutaneous vesicles or bullae, superficial erosions or ulcers, or erythematous macules.

Treatment

- Mild cases undergo spontaneous resolution within weeks to months.
- Corticosteroids (prednisolone, 1 mg/kg daily, by mouth, then reducing to alternate day therapy when control is achieved) may be required in severe cases.

Drug eruptions

Clinical features

- This term is used for any cutaneous manifestation of a reaction to a drug or other chemical gaining access to the body by any route.
- The mechanisms involved are thought to be hypersensitive or allergic but are poorly understood.
- The groups of drugs commonly involved in other species include antibacterial agents (especially penicillins and sulphonamides), phenothiazine-based tranquillisers, non-steroidal anti-inflammatory drugs (especially aspirin and phenylbutazone), diuretics, local anaesthetics and anticonvulsants.
- In horses, antibiotics and potentiated sulphonamides are important. Other drugs that have been implicated include non-steroidal anti-inflammatory drugs, anaesthetic agents and ivermectin. In theory, any drug could be involved.
- A drug eruption may occur after the first exposure to a drug or after many years of use. Signs can appear within 24–48 h of exposure, commonly occur within 1–3 weeks but may be delayed for as long as 2 months.
- Signs: may mimic any skin disease, but certain features should lead to a high index of suspicion, including:
  - Urticaria or angio-oedema, diffuse erythema, bilaterally symmetrical lesions, papular rashes (Figure 4.2), poorly steroid-responsive intense pruritus, sharply demarcated erosions and ulcerations (vasculitis), vesicular and bullous eruptions.

Diagnosis

- Unless considered in the differential diagnosis of skin disease on a frequent basis, drug eruptions will be missed.
- The diagnosis can be based upon ruling out other possibilities, supportive medical history and supportive histopathological changes.

Treatment

- If a drug eruption is suspected, all medication should be withdrawn.
- When some sort of therapy is considered essential, a compound chemically unrelated to current or recently used substances should be chosen.
- Resolution of skin changes usually occurs within 10–14 days but may take months.
- Corticosteroids may provide only minimal relief.
- Future exposure to the suspect drug and related compounds should be avoided.

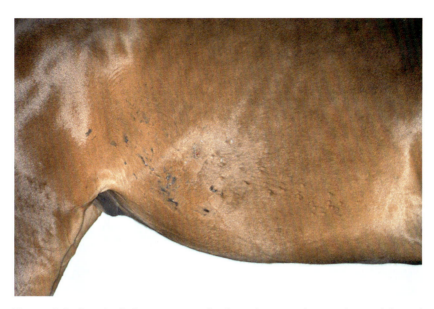

Figure 4.2   Papular lesions, presumed to be a drug eruption, on the caudolateral trunk which appeared within 48 h of administration of penicillin after a surgical procedure.

CONGENITAL AND HEREDITARY CAUSES

Epitheliogenesis imperfecta

Clinical features
- A rare, inherited, congenital cutaneous defect of foals inherited as a single autosomal recessive trait.
- Signs:
  - Lesions are present at birth and consist of sharply demarcated areas where there is an absence of epidermis and skin appendages.
  - Areas usually affected are the distal extremities below carpus and tarsus. Affected areas bleed easily and secondary infection is inevitable with death ensuing from septicaemia.

Diagnosis
- Based on history and clinical signs.
- Unlike epidermolysis bullosa, there is no Nikolsky sign.*
- The preferred site for biopsy is the margin of the lesions.
- Histologically there is complete absence of epidermis and epidermal appendages.

*Nikolsky's sign: superficial epidermis separates when firm, sliding pressure applied to skin.

Treatment and prevention
- There is no effective therapy.
- Dam and sire of affected foals should be removed from breeding programmes.

Epidermolysis bullosa

Clinical features
- This term encompasses a group of hereditary diseases characterised by blister formation following minor trauma. The disease in the horse has been described in the Belgian Draft breed in which it is considered to be an autosomal recessive condition.
- Signs:
  - Lesions are present at birth or occur shortly afterwards and may involve skin, mucocutaneous junctions and oral mucosa.
  - Skin lesions appear as peripherally expanding erosions.
  - Collapsed bullae can frequently be seen in the oral cavity with whitish flaps of mucosa at the edge of lesions.
  - Separation of the hooves at the coronary band is a consistent finding. Dystrophic teeth are common.

Diagnosis
- A positive Nikolsky sign (see footnote on p. 53) can usually be elicited.
- The presence of characteristic lesions in a neonatal Belgian Draft foal is clinically diagnostic.
- Histopathology:
  - Separation is evident at the dermo-epidermal junction, below the basal epithelium, leaving the PAS-positive basement membrane attached to the dermis.

Treatment and prevention
- None is possible. Both sire and dam should be removed from breeding programmes.

Ehlers–Danlos syndrome

Clinical features
- The disease has been reported in Quarter horses and an Arabian crossbred.
- The condition affects collagen synthesis and is apparent at birth or shortly afterwards. It has not been well characterised in the horse to date but is inherited in an autosomal recessive fashion.

- Signs:
  - Lesions may be solitary or multiple and commonly involve the dorsal body surface.
  - Areas of loose skin are found, fairly well demarcated, several inches in diameter.
  - The skin is fragile, tears easily and heals poorly. In good light the centre of lesions appears depressed. Pressure or traction applied at the edge of the lesions may be painful.
  - Occasionally the presenting complaint is haematoma development.
  - Joint hyperextensibility does not appear to be a feature.

Diagnosis
- Characteristic lesions in a young Quarter horse are sufficiently diagnostic.
- Light microscopy may reveal a greatly reduced or absent deep dermal collagen layer, thinning of the dermis, fragmentation and disorientation of collagen fibres.

Treatment and prevention
- There is no treatment.
- Trauma should be minimised.
- Affected and related animals should not be used for breeding.

ENVIRONMENTAL AND NUTRITIONAL CAUSES

Burns

Clinical features
- Burns may result from thermal and chemical insults. Lesions may be classified according to the depth and severity of tissue damage.
- Signs:
  - First-degree burns present with erythema, superficial oedema and marked pain, and resolve after superficial scaling.
  - Second-degree burns show hair loss, superficial blistering and epidermal necrosis with pain. Healing occurs in 7–10 days, with no permanent damage.
  - Third-degree burns have severe blistering with loss of the epidermis and superficial dermis and absence of pain except at the edge of lesions. Healing is slow and scarring ensues with an atrophic epidermis and loss of epidermal appendages.
  - Fourth-degree burns involve loss of full-skin thickness and involve deeper tissues. Serious scarring and impairment of function follows prolonged healing.

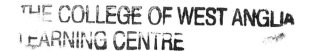

- Assessment of the depth of lesions may be aided by insertion of a needle in the centre of lesions to gauge the presence of pain.
- Considerable loss of plasma protein may accompany second-, third- and fourth-degree burns involving large areas of the body, and secondary infection is common.

Treatment

- Early application of cold water for 20–30 min will limit further tissue damage.
- Intravenous fluid therapy may be required and broad-spectrum anti-biotic cover is indicated.
- Analgesia and sedation may be indicated prior to wound cleansing and debridement.
- Where possible non-adherent semi-occlusive dressings should be applied. Skin grafting may be indicated.
- If burns are extensive or the depth of tissue damage is likely to result in functional impairment, or if there is ocular and lung involvement, then euthanasia may be indicated.

Pressure sores

Clinical features

- The nature of lesions resulting from mechanical damage depends on the nature and duration of frictional forces applied.
  - Sudden or sustained application of a considerable force such as results from a badly fitting harness or tack may result in erosions or ulcerations of the skin, with exudation.
  - Milder pressure or low-grade forces applied repeatedly induce hyperkeratosis, hair loss and callus formation (Figure 4.3). In some cases a dermal reaction occurs, sometimes without overlying hair loss, producing so-called 'corns' or 'sit-fasts'.
  - Prolonged direct pressure, particularly over bony prominences, may result in ischaemic damage and even epidermal sloughing. Incorrectly applied limb bandages are often to blame.
  - Scar tissue with an atrophic epithelium and absence of hair may ensue, or the production of non-pigmented hair if damage is less severe. These changes are typified by saddle sores.

Treatment

- The cause of the damage must be identified and removed.
- In particular, the fit and padding of the saddle should be attended to in cases of dorsal lesions.
- Most minor lesions, including calluses, will resolve given sufficient time.

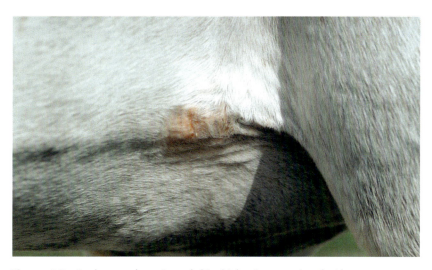

Figure 4.3   Erythema, alopecia and skin thickening associated with pressure sores or 'girth gall'.

- Ischaemic changes and scar formation are permanent.
- Surgery for removal of corns or sit-fasts should be considered a last resort and may cause greater problems.

NEOPLASTIC CAUSES

See Chapter 5.

MISCELLANEOUS DERMATOSES

Actinic dermatoses

Clinical features
- Ultraviolet radiation can damage the skin acutely or chronically.
- Chronic exposure leads to the development of pre-neoplastic and neoplastic diseases.
- Damage resulting from acute exposure can be subdivided into sunburn (Figures 4.4 and 4.5), which results from excessive exposure and is not unexpected, and photosensitisation, which results from normal or minimal exposure.
- Whatever the type of damage, the radiation must be absorbed by the skin and this is facilitated by absence of or a thin haircoat and lack of pigment.

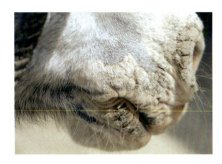

Figure 4.4 Erosion, crusting, fissuring and depigmentation of the muzzle and nares caused by sunburn.

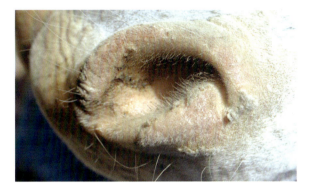

Figure 4.5 Sunburnt external naris showing erythema, scaling and alopecia.

Photosensitisation

Clinical features
- Photosensitisation requires the following:
  - Presence of a photodynamic agent within the skin.
  - Exposure to sufficient amount of certain wavelengths of light.
  - Cutaneous absorption of this ultraviolet radiation.
- Photodynamic agents may be phototoxic or photoallergic.
- Phototoxicity involves no immunological mechanisms, and these agents are capable of causing damage in nearly all animals. Most cases of photosensitisation in horses are of this type.
- Photoallergy requires previous sensitisation and is well recognised in humans, but poorly understood in horses.
- Photodynamic agents may reach the skin by systemic or contact routes.
- Energy is absorbed by the photodynamic molecules and released into the tissues causing damage, primarily to the epidermis and superficial blood vessels.

Systemic photosensitisation

Clinical features

• Primary:
  – This results from ingestion of plants (St John's wort, perennial rye grass) or drugs (phenothiazines, thiazides, methylene blue, sulphonamides, tetracyclines) containing photodynamic agents that are absorbed and reach the skin via the circulation.
• Hepatogenous:
  – Phylloerythrin is a photodynamic agent, which is a metabolite of chlorophyll produced by bacterial fermentation, and is normally excreted in bile. In horses with hepatic disease it may accumulate in the tissues resulting in photosensitisation.
• Signs:
  – Most severe on glabrous non-pigmented skin (lips, eyelids), but can extend to haired regions and to lightly pigmented skin (Figures 4.6 and 4.7).
  – Lesions are variable but may include oedema, erythema and scaling, exudation and crusting, to severe necrosis.
  – Hepatogenous and photoallergic types of photosensitisation tend to occur sporadically, whereas all animals on the pasture are at risk of primary systemic photosensitisation and multiple cases usually occur.

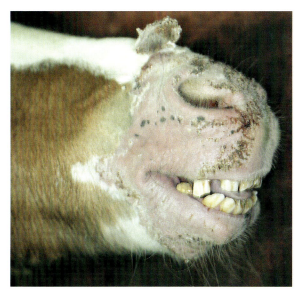

Figure 4.6 Photosensitisation affecting the distal unpigmented skin of the muzzle. A healing lesion.

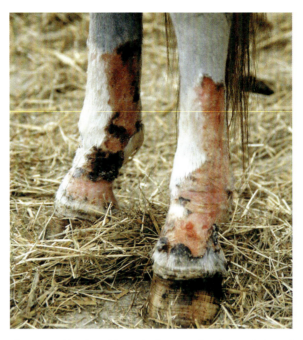

Figure 4.7 Photosensitisation. Alopecia, haemorrhagic exudation, sloughing and ulceration of the non-pigmented distal limbs of a pony out at grass. Several animals in the group were affected, with no evidence of hepatic pathology, indicating primary photosensitisation. (Courtesy of S. C. Shaw.)

Contact photosensitisation

Clinical features

- Most cases have occurred in horses grazing pastures containing clover. Giant hogweed (*Heracleum mantegazzianum*) can also cause contact photosensitisation.
- The incidence of photosensitisation may vary on the same pasture from year to year. It is not understood why clover plants sometimes produce a photodynamic agent.
- Signs:
  - Only areas of contact are involved and lesions are usually restricted to non-pigmented areas of the muzzle and lips and the lower extremities.

Diagnosis of photosensitisation

- Photosensitisation is usually limited to the non-pigmented skin of grazing animals.
- The number of animals involved and distribution of lesions should give a clue to the type of photosensitisation involved (Figure 4.8), but

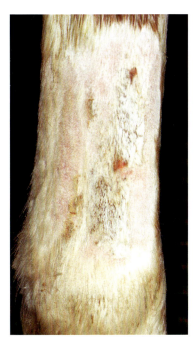

Figure 4.8 Photoaggravated leucocytoclastic vasculitis exhibiting tightly adherent crusts overlying haemorrhagic ulcerated lesions of the metatarsal area.

liver function tests should be run on all cases, since all animals may have been exposed to an agent causing hepatic damage (e.g. ragwort).

Treatment
- Prevent exposure to sunlight by stabling.
- Further exposure to the photodynamic agent should be prevented.
- Corticosteroids used early in the course of the disease will reduce inflammation.
- Non-steroidal anti-inflammatory agents may be indicated.
- Symptomatic topical therapy is also of benefit.

Pastern leucocytoclastic vasculitis

Clinical features
- A specific clinico-pathological entity recognised in horses of either sex, with a predilection in animals with non-pigmented lower limbs and occurring in the summer months in sunny regions.
- Aetiopathogenesis:
  - Poorly understood.
  - Whilst the restriction of lesions to white limbs implicates ultraviolet radiation, no photosensitising process has been determined.

- – Liver function is normal in affected horses and there is no known exposure to photodynamic agents.
        - – An immune-mediated basis is suspected since IgG and/or complement C-3 have been identified in the blood vessel walls of some affected animals.
- Signs:
    - – The condition is usually limited to non-pigmented lower limbs and often only one leg is affected (Figure 4.8), although several may lack pigment.
    - – Occasionally pigmented limbs may be affected.
    - – The lesions affect the medial and lateral aspects of the pastern, are usually multiple and well demarcated.
    - – Initially erythema, oozing and crusting are seen often with marked oedema. Erosions and ulcerations may develop.
    - – Chronically the lesions acquire a rough, warty surface, which is difficult to remove.
    - – Lesions are painful.

Diagnosis
- History; signs – lesions confined to distal non-pigmented skin of limbs.
- Histopathology:
    - – Changes primarily involve the small blood vessels in the superficial dermis.
    - – Leucocytoclastic vasculitis, vessel wall necrosis and thrombosis are seen acutely, and vessel wall thickening and hyalinisation are chronic changes.
    - – Papillomatosis reflects the warty clinical appearance of chronic cases.
    - – A mixed perivascular infiltrate is found in the dermis.
- The major differential diagnosis is photosensitisation, particularly contact type.
    - – Differentiate clinically and by liver function tests.

Treatment
- Stabling the horse prevents further exposure to sunlight; cover with bandages.
- Parenteral corticosteroids are required to reduce inflammation, in relatively high doses (prednisolone 1 mg/kg daily, by mouth, for the first 2 weeks with gradual reduction over the following 2–4 weeks).
- Soaks aid gentle removal of crusts and debris.
- Occasionally recurrence of lesions after withdrawal of steroids requires a further course of therapy, but the condition rarely recurs.

Nodules and swellings

- Nodular diseases form a sizeable component of equine dermatology.
- Important factors to consider are age of onset, speed of onset, breed and sex, coat and/or skin colour, seasonality and history of systemic disease or recent treatment (Figure 5.1).
- Clinical examination is necessary to assess the presence of systemic disease, number of lesions, location on the body surface, signs of injury or trauma, discharge, colour, pain or pruritus. Palpation of lesions is helpful.
- Fungal culture, bacteriology, impression smears of exudate and needle aspirates are often indicated but, in most cases, histopathology is necessary for definitive diagnosis.

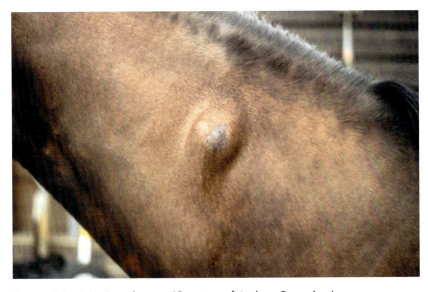

Figure 5.1 Injection abscess. (Courtesy of Andrew Browning.)

PHYSICAL CONDITIONS

Injury

Clinical features
- Bruising: swelling and discoloration of skin.
- Haematoma: firm to hard subcutaneous swelling (Figure 5.2).

Diagnosis
- Diagnostic indicators:
  - History of trauma, physical appearance, skin usually pits on pressure.
- Confirmatory tests:
  - Needle aspirate.
- Differential diagnoses:
  - Abscess, neoplasia, cyst, urticaria.

Treatment and management
- Rest.
- Hot and cold compresses.

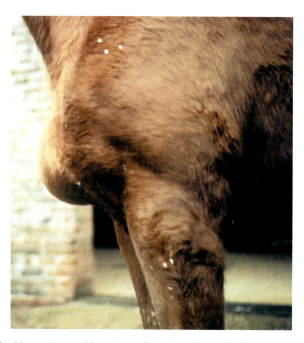

Figure 5.2 Haematoma. (Courtesy of Andrew Browning.)

Bursitis

- Inflammation of a bursa overlying a tendon or joint.

Clinical features
- Swelling in region of a bursa.

Diagnosis
- Diagnostic indicators:
  - History, physical examination.
- Confirmatory tests:
  - Ultrasonography.
  - Needle aspirate. Carefully disinfect skin and employ rigorous aseptic procedures.
- Differential diagnoses:
  - Abscess, bruising, haematoma, calcinosis circumscripta, enlarged joint capsule, neoplasia.

Treatment and management
- Rest.
- Pressure bandages.
- Drainage.
- Glucocorticoids in non-infected cases.
- Surgical drainage or removal.

Hernia (rupture)

- Splitting or tearing of normal muscle sheath or muscle planes allowing protrusion of muscle or abdominal contents – usually scrotal, inguinal or umbilical or wherever muscular injury causes loss of restraint by normal muscle sheath.

Clinical features
- Swelling in areas known to be associated with herniation.

Diagnosis
- Diagnostic indicators:
  - Physical appearance.
- Confirmatory tests:
  - Needle aspirate of gut contents, palpation of guts, ultrasonography, surgical exploration.
- Differential diagnoses:
  - Abscess, haematoma, scirrhous cord, neoplasia.

Treatment and management
- Surgical reduction.

INFECTIOUS CAUSES

Viral infections

Sarcoid

- The most common equine neoplasm.

Clinical features
- Age, breed, sex, colour incidence controversial.
- May occur anywhere, especially on head, legs and ventral trunk (Figure 5.3).
- Sarcoids often multiple.
- Verrucous, fibroblastic, flat (occult), mixed and malevolent forms.
- Cause:
    - Probably papovavirus combined with a genetic predilection; familial tendency may exist.
- Signs:
    - **Verrucous**: slow growing, warty proliferations of skin.
    - **Fibroblastic**: fleshy, proliferative growth, often ulcerative. The most severe form of sarcoid; locally invasive but no metastasis (Figure 5.4).
    - **Flat (occult)**: single or multiple patch of alopecia, scaling and crusting. May stay static and then develop papules or nodules within alopecic areas. Will often become locally aggressive. Verrucous and flat lesions may progress to fibroblastic.
    - **Mixed**: rare – may be transitional between verrucous and fibroblastic.
    - **Malevolent**: multiple very invasive tumours found along lymphatic vessels and local lymph nodes (Figure 5.5).

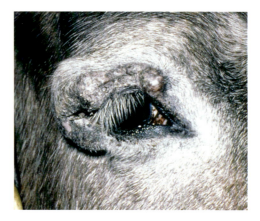

Figure 5.3   Periocular sarcoids. (Courtesy of K. C. Barnett.)

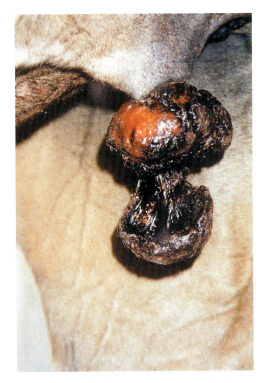

Figure 5.4   Fibroblastic sarcoid. (Courtesy of Pauline Williams.)

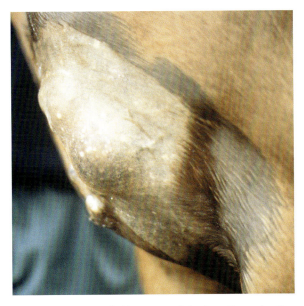

Figure 5.5   Malevolent sarcoid. (Courtesy of Andrew Browning.)

Diagnosis
* Diagnostic indicators:
  – Speed of onset and physical appearance.
* Confirmatory tests:
  – Skin biopsy – **but** may encourage local aggression (contra-indicated in lesions that have not increased in size over a long period).
* Differential diagnoses:
  – **Verrucous**: papillomatosis, squamous cell carcinoma.
  – **Fibroblastic**: squamous cell carcinoma, exuberant granulation tissue, habronemiasis, infectious granulomas, fibroma, fibrosarcoma, neurofibroma, neurofibrosarcoma.
  – **Flat**: dermatophytosis, dermatophilosis, demodicosis, folliculitis, onchocerciasis, alopecia areata.
  – **Malevolent**: lymphangitis.

Treatment and management
Therapeutic approach
* Therapy needs to be tailored to each case depending on availability of treatment, location of tumour, size of tumour, cost and risk. **Specialist advice should be sought**.
  – Ligatures: elastrator rings, Lycra or elastic bands.
  – Conventional surgery: 50% recurrence. Improved success with electrocautery, cryosurgery.
  – *Sarcoid cream (AW4-Ludes*; DC Knottenbelt, Division of Equine Studies, Leahurst, Neston, South Wirral, UK), *arsenic trioxide, podophyllin, 5-fluorouracil. These antineoplastic drugs are applied topically either daily or every 2 days onto small superficial tumours, until resolution of the tumour* (Goodrich et al., 1998; Newton, 2000).
  – Intralesional implants and injections may be effective. Active agents include *cisplatin mixed with sesame seed oil, carboplatin, 5-fluorouracil and bleomycin. Injections of cisplatin are given at 1 mg/cm^3 of tissue 2 weeks apart for four injections.* Cisplatin is mutagenic and carcinogenic and extreme care should be exercised during preparation, handling and administration (Theon, 1998).
  – Immune stimulation: *e.g. BCG (bacille Calmette-Guérin) vaccination.* Administration of BCG may result in severe hypersensitivity and anaphylactic reactions, thus systemic steroids are given prophylactically. Periocular sarcoids are most responsive to this method of treatment (Theon, 1998; Knottenbelt and Kelly, 2000).

    – *Radiation using implanted [22]radon, [198]gold, [226]radium, [60]cobalt or [192]iridium. Good results have been demonstrated using [192]iridium with periocular sarcoids* (Theon, 1998; Newton, 2000). *Radiofrequency hyperthermia and CO_2 laser* reported effective in many cases but expensive.
- Prognosis:
  - Static occult and verrucous: probably best left alone as surgery or biopsy may lead to enlargement and local spread.
  - Fibroblastic will normally need removal.
- Combination therapy improves probability of successful resolution.
- Repeated treatment often needed.

Papillomatosis

Typical

Clinical features
- Common especially in horses younger than 3 years old.
- Incubation period 2–6 months.
- Transmission: direct and indirect.
- Predisposing factors: skin damage, e.g. insect or ectoparasite bite, ultraviolet light.
- Self-limiting.
- Cause:
  - Believed to be a host-specific papovavirus
- Signs:
  - Single or multiple raised, verrucous proliferations of epidermis.
  - Most commonly seen around the eyes, muzzle, lips, distal limbs and external genitalia (Figure 5.6).
  - Variable size: 1 mm to 2 cm.

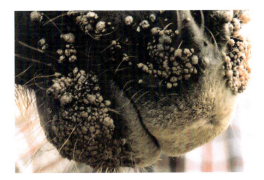

Figure 5.6 Papillomata affecting the muzzle in a 2-year old. (Courtesy of S. Bjornson.)

Diagnosis
- Diagnostic indicators:
  - Age of onset, location on body and physical appearance.
- Confirmatory tests:
  - Skin biopsy, but not usually necessary.
- Differential diagnoses:
  - Sarcoid, viral papular dermatitis, equine molluscum contagiosum.

Treatment and management
Therapeutic approach
- Leave alone.
- Surgery.
- Cryosurgery but may lead to scarring and depigmentation.
- *Topical cytotoxic agents.*
- *Autogenous vaccines but no evidence of efficacy in horses.*
- Prognosis:
  - Spontaneous regression may take from 1 to 6 months.
  - Horses normally develop complete immunity.
- Prophylaxis:
  - Disinfection of premises, avoid contact with affected horses – hard to carry out.

Aural plaques
- Synonyms:
  - Aural flat warts, papillary acanthoma, hyperplastic dermatitis of the ear, squamous papilloma.

Clinical features
- This is a common skin disease of adult horses, caused by a DNA papovavirus.
- No sex or breed predisposition.
- Rare in horses less than 1 year old.
- Transmission may be associated with black fly (*Simulium* spp.).
- Signs:
  - Lesions consist of greyish-white papules, which coalesce to form hyperkeratotic plaques (Figure 5.7) affecting the medial pinnae.
  - There is no associated discomfort in most cases. Occasionally lesions may occur around the anus, vulva and inguinal regions.

Diagnosis
- Diagnostic indicators:
  - Age of onset and physical appearance.

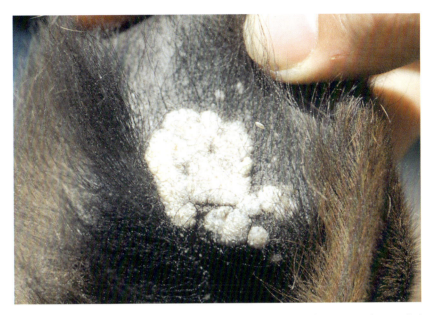

Figure 5.7 Aural plaques. Depigmented hyperkeratotic plaques on the medial surface of the pinna.

- Confirmatory tests:
  - Histopathology of shave skin biopsy specimens but not usually necessary.
- Differential diagnoses:
  - None.

Treatment and management
- No effective treatment available
- Prognosis:
  - Lesions tend to persist indefinitely.

Viral papular dermatitis

Clinical features
- Cause:
  - An unclassified poxvirus.
- Signs:
  - Initially – small non-pruritic papules on the trunk, neck and legs.
  - After 7 days – crusting.
  - After about 14 days – annular alopecia and scaling.

Diagnosis
- Diagnostic indicators:
  - Speed of onset and physical appearance.
- Confirmatory tests:
  - Virus isolation and skin biopsy.
- Differential diagnoses:
  - Staphylococcal folliculitis, dermatophilosis, dermatophytosis, demodicosis.

Treatment and management
- No specific treatment.
- Prognosis.
  - Spontaneous remission usually occurs within 4–6 weeks.

Equine molluscum contagiosum

Clinical features
- Cause:
  - An unclassified poxvirus.
- Signs:
  - Multiple waxy papules which may coalesce and produce a caseous discharge.
  - Lesions occur on penis, prepuce, scrotum, mammary glands, thighs, axillae and muzzle.

Diagnosis
- Diagnostic indicators:
  - Location of lesions and physical appearance.
- Confirmatory tests:
  - Skin biopsies.
- Differential diagnoses:
  - Papillomatosis, viral papular dermatitis

Treatment and management
No specific treatment.
- Prognosis:
  - Regression may take years.

Bacterial infections

Folliculitis and furunculosis

See Chapter 3.

Cellulitis

Clinical features
- Rare, no age or sex predilection.
- Poorly defined, severe, deep, suppurative infection involving the subcutaneous tissues.
- Cause:
  - Staphylococci or anaerobic bacteria often involved.
  - All reported cases of staphylococcal cellulitis have occurred in Thoroughbred racehorses in active training.
  - No obvious association with trauma or infections.
- Signs:
  - Severe and painful swelling of one (often hind) limb with extreme lameness.
  - Pyrexia, tachycardia and distress.
  - Complications include necrosis, sloughing, laminitis of affected or contralateral limb, osteomyelitis and bacteraemia.

Diagnosis
- Diagnostic indicators:
  - Sudden onset of severe lameness and physical appearance.

Treatment
Therapeutic approach
- Prolonged systemic antibiotics until healing has occurred.
  - If mild, trimethoprim sulphadiazine, 15–30 mg/kg twice daily, by mouth or *procaine penicillin, 15–20 mg/kg twice daily, intramuscularly.*
  - If severe, *gentamicin, 6 mg/kg intravenously, once daily, procaine penicillin, 20 mg/kg twice daily, intramuscularly (benzylpenicillin can be used intravenously if intramuscular injections are not well tolerated).*
  - Ceftiofur (Excenel, Pfizer Animal Health), 2 mg/kg once daily.
  - *Oral enrofloxacin can be used for longer-term therapy (but not in immature horses). Baytril 10% Oral Solution (Bayer) is used at 5.0–7.5 mg/kg once daily. This is a poultry preparation not licensed for the horse.*
- Non-steroidal anti-inflammatory drugs.
- Support bandages on the affected and contralateral limb.
- Prognosis:
  - Guarded.

Abscesses

Clinical features
- Localised, fluctuant to solid lesions consisting of dead cells, debris and liquefied tissue.
- Contamination of skin wounds, vaccination sites.
- Cause:
  - *Corynebacterium pseudotuberculosis, Clostridium* spp. and staphylococci are often involved.
- Signs:
  - Circumscribed, subcutaneous accumulations of pus.

Diagnosis
- Diagnostic indicators:
  - Clinical signs.
- Confirmatory tests:
  - Stained smears of needle aspirate, bacterial culture.
  - Ultrasound.
- Differential diagnoses:
  - Cysts, haematomas, mycetomas, neoplasia.

Treatment
Therapeutic approach
- Surgical drainage and debridement.
- Flushing and packing with topical antimicrobial agents.
- Systemic antibiotics based on sensitivity testing; not before the abscess matures.
- If *Clostridium* spp. involved, use aggressive drainage and high-dose antimicrobial therapy, *e.g. 40 mg/kg benzyl penicillin twice to four times daily with clostridial myositis.*
- Prognosis:
  - Usually good. If involving *Clostridium* spp. or in a site of poor drainage, poor prognosis.
- Prophylaxis:
  - General hygiene.

Ulcerative lymphangitis

Clinical features
- Very rare.
- Contamination of skin wounds.
- Transmission by direct contact or insect vectors.
- Cause:

– Usually *Corynebacterium pseudotuberculosis* and/or *Pseudomonas aeruginosa*.
• Signs:
 – Painful, discharging nodules on distal hind limbs – unilateral or bilateral.
 – Pyrexia common.
 – Regional lymphatics may show enlargement, hardening and ulceration leading to lameness and debility.
 – New lesions may continue to appear for years.
 – Sometimes fatal.

Diagnosis
• Diagnostic indicators:
 – Clinical signs.
• Confirmatory tests:
 – Stained smears and skin biopsies for culture and histopathology.
• Differential diagnoses:
 – Sporotrichosis, actinomycosis, nocardiosis, mycobacterial infections.

Treatment
Therapeutic approaches
• Surgical drainage, hydrotherapy, exercise.
• *Prolonged high doses of procaine penicillin (15–50 mg/kg twice daily by intramuscular injection).*
• *Autogenous bacterins* – of doubtful efficacy.
• Prognosis:
 – Cure is unlikely in the later stages, when fibrosis is present.
• Prophylaxis:
 – Good hygiene and management; early wound treatment and effective insect control.

Bacterial mycetoma

Clinical features
• Chronic subcutaneous infection where bacteria are present in tissues as granules or grains.
• Cause:
 – Actinomycotic mycetoma: *Actinobacillus*, *Nocardia* and *Actinomyces* spp.
 – Other bacteria, e.g. staphylococci (botryomycosis), *Pseudomonas* spp.
• Signs:
 – Ulcerative nodules (Figure 5.8) with draining tracts and usually tissue granules (grains).

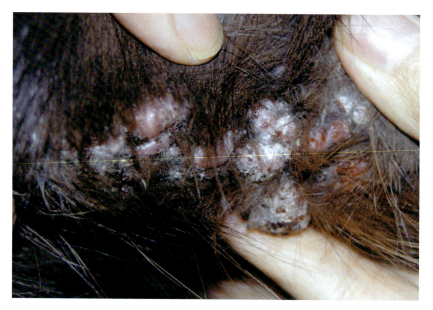

Figure 5.8   Nodular lesions of botryomycosis (*S. aureus*), 1–2 cm diameter, with alopecia and crusting, along the mandible of a horse.

Diagnosis
- Diagnostic indicators:
  - Clinical signs.
- Confirmatory tests:
  - Bacterial culture, stained smears of needle aspirates and skin biopsies with special stains.
- Differential diagnoses:
  - Fungal granulomas, habronemiasis, exuberant granulation tissue, neoplasia.

Treatment
Therapeutic approach
- Prolonged antibiotics based on sensitivity; radical surgical excision.
- Antibacterials include:
  - If mild, trimethoprim sulphadiazine, 15–30 mg/kg twice daily, by mouth or *procaine penicillin, 10–20 mg/kg once daily, intramuscularly.*
  - Ceftiofur (Excenel, Pfizer Animal Health), 2 mg/kg once daily.
  - *Oral enrofloxacin can be used for longer-term therapy (but not in immature horses). Baytril 10% Oral Solution (Bayer) is used at 5.0–7.5 mg/kg once daily.* This is a poultry preparation not licensed for the horse.

Tuberculosis

Clinical features
- Skin involvement very rare.
- Cause:
  - *Mycobacterium intracellulare*, *M. avium* and *M. smegmatis*
- Signs:
  - Scaling, alopecia, nodules and ulceration, abscess formation; systemic signs include fever, diarrhoea, weight loss and lymphadenopathy.

Diagnosis
- Diagnostic indicators:
  - History of contact with infected animal, physical examination, clinical signs, radiography.
- Confirmatory tests:
  - Mycobacterial culture, serology and skin biopsies with special stains. Tuberculin tests are not useful as 70% of normal horses show positive intradermal reactions to purified mammalian and avian tuberculin.

Treatment and prognosis
- Euthanasia. Infection is almost invariably fatal but recovery from an abscess infected with the atypical mycobacterial species, *M. smegmatis*, has been reported (Booth and Wattret, 2000).

FUNGAL INFECTIONS

Dermatophytosis

See Chapter 3.

Fungal mycetoma

Clinical features
- Chronic subcutaneous infection where fungi present in tissues as granules or grains.
- Cause:
  - Eumycotic mycetoma: soil-living species *Curvularia geniculata*, *Pseudoallescheria boydii*.
- Signs:
  - Chronic subcutaneous nodules, often ulcerative with draining tracts and tissue granules or grains in discharge (Figure 5.9).

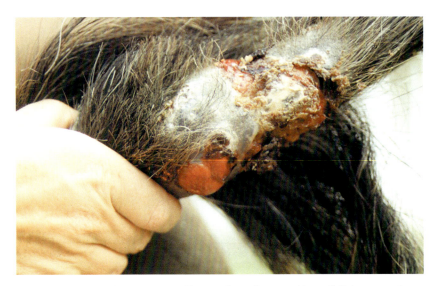

Figure 5.9   Fungal mycetoma, affecting the tail, caused by soil-living organisms.

Diagnosis
- Diagnostic indicators:
  - Clinical signs.
- Confirmatory tests:
  - Stained smears of needle aspirates, fungal culture.
- Differential diagnoses:
  - Actinomycotic mycetoma, bacterial and fungal pseudomycetoma.

Treatment
Therapeutic approach
- Surgical removal.
- Iodides.
  - *Sodium iodide: 50 mg/kg intravenously as 3.5% solution in normal saline. Two doses, 3–7 days apart.*
  - *Potassium iodide: 10 g per 450 kg twice daily by mouth for 10 days or until iodism occurs.*

Signs of iodide toxicity: dry scurfy skin, watery eyes and nose, enlarged thyroid gland, depression, weight loss, anorexia, fever, coughing, alopecia.
- Prognosis:
  - Guarded. Medical therapy often unsuccessful.
- Prophylaxis:
  - Good hygiene and management; early wound treatment and effective insect control.

Phaeohyphomycosis (chromomycosis)

Clinical features
- Usually occurs through wound contamination.
- Cause:
  - *Drechslera spicifera*, *Alternaria alternata* and other ubiquitous pigmented (dematiaceous) saprophytic fungi.
- Signs:
  - Plaques, papules and pustules.
  - Slow-growing, solitary or multiple, subcutaneous masses often ulcerated.
  - Found on neck, body, legs.

Diagnosis
- Diagnostic indicators:
  - History and clinical signs.
- Confirmatory tests:
  - Smears of discharge (*Drechslera* organised in septate hyphae, not into granules), skin biopsy and fungal culture.
- Differential diagnoses:
  - Collagenolytic granuloma, mycetomas.

Treatment
Therapeutic approach
- Systemic iodides:
  - *Sodium iodide: 50 mg/kg intravenously as 3.5% solution in normal saline. Two doses 3–7 days apart.*
  - *Potassium iodide: 10 g per 450 kg twice daily by mouth for 10 days or until iodism occurs.*

Signs of iodide toxicity: dry scurfy skin, watery eyes and nose, enlarged thyroid gland, depression, weight loss, anorexia, fever, coughing, alopecia.
- *Ketoconazole (Nizoral, Janssen-Cilag): 30 mg/kg once daily or twice daily. Itraconazole (Sporanox, Janssen-Cilag): 3 mg/kg twice daily for < 2 months.*
- *Amphotericin B (Fungizone, Squibb): 0.3 mg/kg per day in 1 litre of 5% dextrose given slowly intravenously. Daily dose increased to a maximum of 1 mg/kg for < 30 days.*
- Prophylaxis:
  - Good hygiene and management; early wound treatment and effective insect control.

Sporotrichosis

Clinical features
- Rare; zoonotic; usually occurs through wound contamination.
- Only one horse in a herd is usually infected.

- Cause:
  - *Sporothrix schenckii,* ubiquitous saprophytic fungus.
- Signs:
  - Hard subcutaneous nodules that ulcerate and produce creamy pus.
  - Lymphatics often affected on medial legs.
  - Sometimes systemic involvement.

Diagnosis
- Diagnostic indicators:
  - History and clinical signs.
- Confirmatory tests:
  - Stained smears of discharge, fungal culture, serology.
- Differential diagnoses:
  - Mycetomas, phaeohyphomycosis, abscess and neoplasia.

Treatment and management
Therapeutic approach
- Surgical removal of masses.
- Systemic iodides:
  - *Sodium iodide: 50 mg/kg intravenously as 3.5% solution in normal saline. Two doses 3–7 days apart.*
  - *Potassium iodide: 10 g per 450 kg twice daily by mouth for 10 days or until iodism occurs.*

Signs of iodide toxicity: dry scurfy skin, watery eyes and nose, enlarged thyroid gland, depression, weight loss, anorexia, fever, coughing, alopecia.
- *Ketoconazole (Nizoral, Janssen-Cilag): 30 mg/kg once daily or twice daily. Itraconazole (Sporanox, Janssen-Cilag): 3 mg/kg twice daily for < 2 months.*
- *Amphotericin B (Fungizone, Squibb): 0.3 mg/kg per day in 1 litre of 5% dextrose given slowly iv. Daily dose increased to a maximum of 1 mg/kg for <30 days.*
- Prognosis:
  - Lesions should regress after 3–4 weeks of antifungal therapy.
- Prophylaxis:
  - Good hygiene and management; early wound treatment and effective insect control.

PARASITIC INFESTATIONS

Hypodermiasis

Clinical features
- Eradicated from UK but may occur in imported horses.

- Anaphylaxis reported following death or rupture of larvae.
- Cattle are primary hosts.
- Seasonal incidence around spring.
- Cause
  - Infestation by larvae of warble fly (*Hypoderma bovis, H. lineatum*).
- Signs:
  - Subcutaneous nodules and cysts over dorsum.
  - Opening or breathing pore frequently develops.
  - Sometimes pruritic.

Diagnosis
- Diagnostic indicators:
  - Imported.
  - History and clinical signs.
- Confirmatory tests:
  - Demonstration of larvae.
- Differential diagnoses:
  - Infectious granulomas, cysts, neoplasia, collagenolytic granuloma.

Treatment and management
Therapeutic approach
- Removal of larva.
- Surgical removal of entire nodule.
- Prognosis:
  - Fair.
- Prophylaxis:
  - Effective insect control.

Demodicosis

Clinical features
- Rare.
- Cause:
  - *Demodex equi* and *D. caballi*.
  - Immunosuppression may be a factor.
- Signs:
  - Alopecia, scaling and variable pyoderma (Figure 5.10).
  - Nodular form is less common.

Diagnosis
- Diagnostic indicators:
  - History and clinical signs.

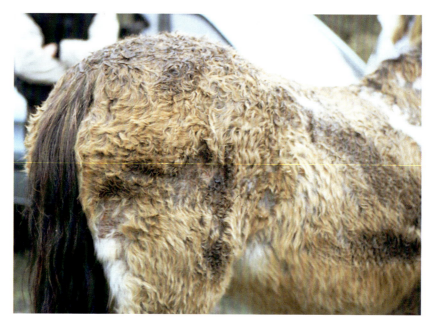

Figure 5.10   Demodicosis and folliculitis associated with alopecia, erythema and excoriation in a 23-year-old pony.

- Confirmatory tests:
  - Demonstration of mites in skin scrapings or material expressed from nodules.
- Differential diagnoses:
  - Infectious granulomas, hypodermiasis, cysts, neoplasia, collageno-lytic granuloma.

Treatment and management
Therapeutic approach
- Treat only if symptomatic; may regress without treatment.
- Identification and correction of underlying immunosuppressive factors or concurrent disease.
- *Topical acaricides or oral ivermectin may be effective.*
- Amitraz may cause death in horses and is completely contraindicated.
- Prognosis:
  - Fair to guarded depending on underlying factors.

Habronemiasis

See Chapter 4.

NEOPLASIA

Sarcoid and papillomatosis

See viral nodules and swellings in the section on Infectious causes.

Melanoma

Clinical features
- Very common, especially on grey and white coated horses.
- About 67% of cases malignant.
- Rarely seen in horses under 6 years old.
- No sex predilection.
- Signs:
  - Small hard tumours in subcutis.
  - Slowly increase in size but rapidly fatal once vital organs are involved.
  - Anus, vulva and tail commonly involved (Figures 5.11 and 5.12). Less commonly male genitalia, limbs, ears, eyelids and neck.

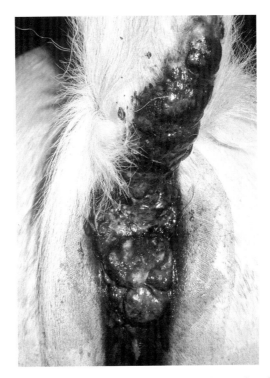

Figure 5.11 Melanotic tumours around the anus, vulva and under the tail of a mare with melanoma.

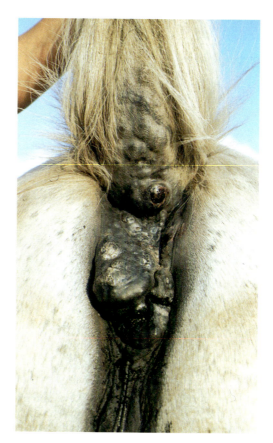

Figure 5.12 Amelanotic melanomas affecting the perineum and undersurface of the tail.

- Sometimes ulcerative with a black discharge.
- May be associated with dystocia or problems in defecation.

Diagnosis
- Diagnostic indicators:
  - History and clinical signs.
- Confirmatory tests:
  - Stained smears of fine needle aspirate, skin biopsy.
- Differential diagnoses:
  - Melanocytic tumours recently differentiated into four syndromes:
    - Melanocytic nevus.
    - Anaplastic malignant melanoma.
    - Dermal melanoma.
    - Dermal melanomatosis.

Treatment
Therapeutic approach
- Radical surgical excision, cryotherapy.
- *Cimetidine at 4 mg/kg three times daily by mouth for 3 months; if tumour regresses continue at 2.5 mg/kg by mouth* (Theon, 1998).
- *Intralesional cisplatin, 1 mg/cm^3 of tissue every second week for four treatments.*
- Prognosis:
  - Poor.

Cutaneous lymphoma

Clinical features
- Rare.
- Usually forms part of multicentric, alimentary or thymic malignant lymphoma.
- May arise at any site in the body where there is lymphoreticular tissue.
- Accounts for only 1–3% of all tumours but is one of the most common causes of neoplasia-associated deaths in horses.
- Seen in all ages.
- Possibly more common in males than females.
- Primary cutaneous form recently reported in the UK.
- Signs:
  - Multifocal, firm subcutaneous nodules without inflammation or alopecia.
  - Systemic signs including weight loss and diarrhoea.
  - Clinical course usually rapid and disease fatal.

Diagnosis
- Diagnostic indicators:
  - History and clinical signs.
- Confirmatory tests:
  - Skin biopsy and immunohistochemical staining.
- Differential diagnoses:
  - Collagenolytic granuloma, sterile panniculitis, sarcoid, fibroma, mastocytosis, melanoma, squamous cell carcinoma, amyloidosis.

Treatment
Therapeutic approaches
- Euthanasia in multicentric, alimentary or thymic forms.
- *Glucocorticoids, progestagens and androgens have been used successfully in primary cutaneous form. Methotrexate 100 mg once daily every 4 days combined with dexamethasone said to have benefit in some horses* (Johnson, 1998). *A single intralesional injection of betamethasone (Betsolan injection,*

Schering-Plough) coupled with megestrol acetate tablets (Ovarid, Schering-Plough), 0.2 mg/kg daily by mouth for 8 days was effective in a single case (Littlewood et al., 1995).
- *Cyclophosphamide 300 mg/m² body surface.*
- *Cytosine arabinoside (200–300 mg/m² intramuscularly once every 1–2 weeks), chlorambucil (20 mg/m² by mouth every 2 weeks alternated with the cytosine arabinoside) and prednisolone (1–2 mg/kg by mouth every 48 h). If remission has not occurred within 4 weeks, treatment with vincristine (0.5 mg/m² intravenously once weekly) is incorporated into the protocol* (Couto, 1994).
- *Immunotherapy with vaccinia virus-infected autologous tumour cell.*
- Prognosis:
  - Poor.

Squamous cell carcinoma

Clinical features
- Second most common equine tumour (accounts for 20% of all equine tumours).
- Most common periocular and periadnexal tumour, and most common tumour of the stomach.
- Mean age incidence of 12 years; males may be predisposed; no breed predilection.
- Associated with chronic exposure of unpigmented, poorly haired skin to ultraviolet light.
- Smegma implicated in development of penile and preputial lesions.
- Signs:
  - Head (conjunctiva and eyelids), mucocutaneous junctions and external genitalia are common sites (Figure 5.13).
  - Lesions usually proliferative with secondary ulceration; sometimes primarily erosive.
  - May present as chronic non-healing ulcer.
  - Haemorrhage and secondary infection may occur.

Diagnosis
- Diagnostic indicators:
  - History and clinical signs.
- Confirmatory tests:
  - Histopathological examination of excised material.
- Differential diagnoses:
  - Habronemiasis, exuberant granulation tissue, fibroblastic sarcoid and other cutaneous neoplasms.

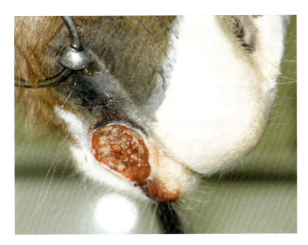

Figure 5.13   Squamous cell carcinoma. An ulcerated mass on the non-pigmented lower lip of a 25-year-old horse. Regional lymphadenopathy was also present. (Courtesy of M. J. Brearley.)

Treatment
Therapeutic approach
- Wide surgical excision, cryosurgery.
- Radiotherapy – brachytherapy using radioisotopes including gold, strontium, iridium.
- Chemotherapy: *intralesional cisplatin at 1 mg/cm^3 of tissue 2 weeks apart for four injections and 5-fluorouracil; topical 5-fluorouracil daily for 3–4 months until tumour regression.*
- *Intralesional BCG also reported to work* (McCalla et al., 1992).
- Lasers may reduce recurrence and spread.
- Prognosis:
  – Locally aggressive and may later spread to lymph nodes and lungs.
  – Penile and preputial lesions tend to be more aggressive.

IMMUNE-MEDIATED CAUSES

Erythema multiforme

See Chapter 3.

Urticaria

See Chapter 2.

Cutaneous amyloidosis

Clinical features
- Affects skin and upper respiratory tract. No age, breed or sex predilection.
- Slow, progressive development of lesions.
- Cause:
  - Unknown.
- Signs:
  - Multiple, hard, non-painful cutaneous nodules, papules and plaques 0.5–10 cm in diameter.
  - Overlying skin usually normal.
  - Anterior parts of the body often affected.
  - Initial lesions sometimes resemble urticaria and may resolve spontaneously.
  - Dyspnoea may result when involvement of nasal mucosa is severe.
  - Internal organs rarely involved.

Diagnosis
- Diagnostic indicators:
  - History and clinical signs.
- Confirmatory tests:
  - Skin biopsies with special stains (Congo red, crystal violet, thioflavin T).
- Differential diagnoses:
  - Neoplasia, collagenolytic granuloma, mastocytosis, mycetoma.

Treatment
Therapeutic approach
- None likely to be effective.
- Tracheotomy to ensure patent airway.
- May be best not to breed from affected horses (some human forms have genetic basis).
- Prognosis:
  - Disease often prolonged and progressive.

MISCELLANEOUS

Collagenolytic granuloma

Synonyms
- Eosinophilic granuloma, nodular necrobiosis with collagen degeneration, acute collagen necrosis.

Clinical features

- Common; no age, breed or sex predilection.
- Occurs mostly in spring and summer.
- May resolve spontaneously but recurrence common.
- Cause:
  - Unknown cause and pathogenesis – possible multiple aetiology including hypersensitivity to insect bites.
- Signs:
  - Single or multiple dermal lesions (Figure 5.14), variable diameter (0.5–10 cm).
  - Often in saddle area but also neck and flanks, occasionally whole body surface.
  - Rounded, well circumscribed, firm, non-alopecic, non-ulcerative, non-painful and non-pruritic.
  - Overlying skin surface and hair usually normal unless traumatised.
  - Mineralisation in chronic lesions.

Diagnosis

- Diagnostic indicators:
  - History and clinical signs.
- Confirmatory tests:
  - Stained smears of needle aspirate, skin biopsy.

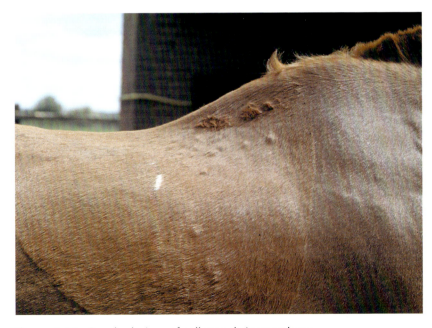

Figure 5.14 Papular lesions of collagenolytic granuloma.

- Differential diagnoses:
    - Hypodermiasis, viral papular dermatitis, unilateral papular dermatosis, staphylococcal folliculitis and furunculosis, dermatophytosis, neoplasia, calcinosis circumscripta.

Treatment
Therapeutic approach
- Leave alone.
- Modify saddle padding for localised saddle patch lesions.
- Surgical excision – if single or few lesions.
- Systemic, intralesional or sublesional injections of glucocorticoid.
    - Prednisolone: 1 mg/kg once daily by mouth for 2–3 weeks.
    - *Dexamethasone (Opticorten, Novartis): 0.1 mg/kg once daily by mouth as a loading dose then 0.04 mg/kg or less every 72–96 h for 2–3 weeks.*
    - *Methylprednisolone acetate: 5–10 mg per lesion. Repeat after 2 weeks if necessary.*
    - *Triamcinolone acetonide: 3–5 mg per lesion. No more than 20 mg per horse. Repeat after 2 weeks if necessary.*
- Prognosis:
    - Glucocorticoids probably ineffective in later stages after mineralisation.
    - Treatment unlikely to produce permanent remission.

Axillary nodular necrosis

Clinical features
- Rare condition affecting mature horses.
- Working and non-working horses.
- Only one out of a group affected.
- Cause:
    - Unknown.
- Signs:
    - Usually unilateral.
    - Round, firm, well-circumscribed, non-alopecic, non-ulcerative, non-painful, non-pruritic subcutaneous nodules near girth and axillae.
    - Single or multiple.
    - Size of nodules varies between 1 and 5 cm.

Diagnosis
- Diagnostic indicators:
    - History and clinical signs.

- Confirmatory tests:
  - Stained smears of needle aspirate, skin biopsy, bacterial and fungal culture to rule out differentials.
- Differential diagnoses:
  - Collagenolytic granuloma, pressure sores, infectious granuloma, cutaneous amyloidosis, mastocytosis, lymphosarcoma and other neoplastic conditions.

Treatment
Therapeutic approach
- Surgical excision or sublesional glucocorticoids.
  - *Methylprednisolone acetate: 5–10 mg per lesion. Repeat after 2 weeks if necessary.*
- Prognosis:
  - Uncertain.
  - Variable response to glucocorticoids.

Mastocytosis

Clinical features
- Uncommon; reactive or hyperplastic process rather than neoplastic; metastasis not reported. No spontaneous regression.
- Signs: two forms are recognised.
  - Usually a single cutaneous nodule (Figure 5.15) often on the head. Size range from 2 to 20 cm diameter. Surface may be normal, hairless or ulcerated.

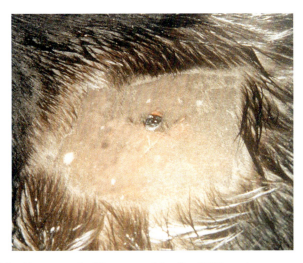

Figure 5.15 Mastocytosis. (Courtesy of Pauline Williams.)

- Less commonly, swelling of a lower extremity often below carpus or hock, not associated with lameness. May become mineralised.
- May also present at birth with multiple masses, which may regress and reform.

Diagnosis
- Diagnostic indicators:
  - History and clinical signs.
- Confirmatory tests:
  - Stained smears of needle aspirate, skin biopsy.
- Differential diagnoses:
  - Collagenolytic granuloma, neoplasia, cutaneous amyloidosis, mycetomas

Treatment and management
Therapeutic approach
- Surgical excision.
- Systemic or intralesional glucocorticoids.
  - Prednisolone: 1 mg/kg once daily by mouth for 2–3 weeks.
  - *Dexamethasone (Opticorten, Novartis): 0.1 mg/kg once daily by mouth for 2–3 weeks.*
  - *Methylprednisolone acetate: 5–10 mg per lesion. Repeat after 2 weeks if necessary.*
  - *Triamcinolone acetonide: 3–5 mg per lesion. No more than 20 mg per horse. Repeat after 2 weeks if necessary.*
- Radiotherapy.

Unilateral papular dermatosis

Clinical features
- Uncommon.
- Cause:
  - Multifactorial aetiology including contact with bedding, insect bites, peripheral neuropathy, infectious agent.
- Signs:
  - Unilateral papules.
  - Usually neither pruritic nor painful.
  - No systemic illness.

Diagnosis
- Diagnostic indicators:
  - Characteristic unilateral presentation and skin biopsy.

- Confirmatory tests:
  - None.
- Differential diagnoses:
  - Collagenolytic granuloma, viral papular dermatitis, staphylococcal folliculitis and furunculosis, dermatophytosis, neoplasia, calcinosis circumscripta.

Treatment and management
Therapeutic approach
- Leave alone.
- Systemic glucocorticoids:
  - Prednisolone: 1 mg/kg once daily by mouth for 2–3 weeks.
  - *Dexamethasone (Opticorten, Novartis): 0.1 mg/kg once daily by mouth for 2–3 weeks.*
Prognosis
- Some cases resolve after a few weeks or months.
- Sometimes recurrent.
- Glucocorticoids may hasten recovery.
- Prophylaxis:
  - Insect control.

Generalised (systemic) granulomatous disease

See Chapter 3.

CYSTS

- Epithelium-lined cavities containing fluid or solid material.
- Smooth, well-circumscribed, fluctuant to solid mass.
- Uncommon.

Epidermoid cyst

- Synonyms: atheroma, epithelial inclusion cyst.

Clinical features
- Subcutaneous nodule found unilaterally (rarely bilateral) in or over false nostril (false nostril cyst); this may be congenital but not noticed until horse is 3–6 months old.
- Does not usually cause respiratory noise or obstruction.
- May occur around base of the ear and may produce mucoid secretion (dentigerous cyst).

- Cause:
  - Congenital or acquired through occlusion of hair follicle or trau-matic implantation of epidermis.
- Signs:
  - Solitary or multiple.
  - Well-circumscribed, firm, non-alopecic, non-ulcerative, non-painful and non-pruritic nodule.
  - Progressive exfoliation of keratinised material leads to enlargement of cyst.
  - Overlying skin surface and hair usually normal unless traumatised.

Diagnosis
- Diagnostic indicators:
  - History and clinical signs.
  - Needle aspirate – no evidence of pus.
- Confirmatory tests:
  - Skin biopsy.
- Differential diagnoses:
  - Abscess, foreign body, fistula, other cysts, neoplasia.

Treatment and management
Therapeutic approach
- Leave.
- Surgical excision.
- Prognosis:
  - Unlikely to resolve without therapy.

Dermoid cyst

Clinical features
- Congenital or hereditary.
- Age range of 6 months to 9 years.
- Wall contains epidermal appendages.
- Lumen contains hair and secretions from sebaceous and sweat glands in addition to keratin.
- Cause:
  - Embryonic displacement of ectoderm into subcutis.
- Signs:
  - Solitary or multiple.
  - Well-circumscribed, firm, non-alopecic, non-ulcerative, non-painful and non-pruritic nodule.
  - Overlying skin surface and hair usually normal unless traumatised.
  - Dorsal midline between withers and rump.

Diagnosis
- Diagnostic indicators:
  - History and clinical signs.
  - Needle aspirate.
- Confirmatory tests:
  - Skin biopsy.
- Differential diagnoses:
  - Abscess, foreign body, other cysts, neoplasia.

Treatment
Therapeutic approach
- Leave.
- Surgical excision.
- Prognosis:
  - Unlikely to resolve without therapy.

Conchal (periauricular) cyst

Clinical features
- Rare; no age, breed or sex predilection.
- Cause:
  - Developmental defect.
- Signs:
  - Fluctuating non-painful swelling.
  - Solitary, occurs near base of the ear, may discharge a sero-mucoid secretion.

Diagnosis
- Diagnostic indicators:
  - History and clinical signs.
  - Needle aspirate.
- Confirmatory tests:
  - Skin biopsy.
- Differential diagnoses:
  - Abscess, foreign body, fistula, dentigerous cysts, neoplasia.

Treatment
Therapeutic approach
- Leave.
  - Surgical excision.
- Prognosis:
  - Unlikely to resolve without therapy.

Calcinosis circumscripta

Synonym: tumoral calcinosis.

Clinical features
- Formation of calcified granular deposits in subcutis.
- Most commonly reported in young male Standardbreds.
- Age incidence typically 12–18 months.
- Cause:
  - Unknown. May be associated with prolonged or repeated trauma or with error in phosphorus metabolism inherited as an autosomal recessive gene.
- Signs:
  - Hard, well-circumscribed, subcutaneous nodules about 3–12 cm in diameter.
  - Non-painful and non-pruritic.
  - Single or multiple.
  - Overlying skin normal.
  - Frequently occurs near joints or tendon sheaths especially over lateral stifle (unilateral or bilateral).
  - No lameness associated.

Diagnosis
- Diagnostic indicators:
  - History and clinical signs.
- Confirmatory tests:
  - Skin biopsies and radiography.
- Differential diagnoses:
  - Neoplasia, collagenolytic and infectious granulomata, mastocytosis, amyloidosis.

Treatment
Therapeutic approach
  - Leave alone.
  - Surgical excision.
- Prognosis:
  - Postoperative wound breakdown is common.

Exuberant granulation tissue

Synonyms: proud flesh, excessive granulation tissue.

Clinical features
- Overgrowth above adjacent epithelium of normal granulation tissue following injury or trauma.
- Often associated with chemical irritants, bacterial infection or contamination with debris such as hair, dirt, gravel, buried sutures and inappropriate wound management.
- Cause:
  - Unknown.
- Signs:
  - Proliferation of granulation tissue with no healing or epithelium production.
  - Tissue is pink to red, firm and granular.
  - Frequently occurs on distal limbs.

Diagnosis
- Diagnostic indicators:
  - History, clinical signs, lesion location.
- Confirmatory tests:
  - Skin biopsies.
- Differential diagnoses:
  - Fibroblastic sarcoid, habronemiasis, squamous cell carcinoma, infectious granulomata.

Treatment and management
Therapeutic approach
- Surgical trimming or excision of the exuberant tissue and removal of a narrow strip (2 mm) of the surrounding skin to reinitiate healing and promote re-epithelialisation. Wounds should be covered and kept moist with the use of hydrogels and hydrocolloids.
- Coupled with limb immobilisation, control of infection and local glucocorticoid therapy; prevent self-trauma.
- Skin grafting will accelerate healing and reduce scar formation.
- Chemical cauterisation should be avoided.
- Prognosis:
  - Guarded. Improved by early grafting.
- Prophylaxis:
  - Good hygiene and wound care.

Nodular panniculitis

Clinical features
- Rare inflammatory condition affecting subcutaneous fat.
- No age, breed or gender predilection.
- Cause:
  - Multifactorial: skin infections, immune-mediated conditions (lupus, drug eruption, vasculitis), physicochemical factors (trauma, pressure, cold, foreign body, injection of bulky, oily or insoluble liquids), systemic disease (pancreatitis), glucocorticoid therapy, nutritional (vitamin E) deficiency, enteropathy.
  - Sometimes idiopathic.
- Signs:
  - Single or multiple nodules affecting trunk, neck and proximal limbs.
  - Variable pain and texture.
  - Ulceration and draining tracts may develop.
  - Variable systemic signs – anorexia, pyrexia, lethargy, depression.

Diagnosis
- Diagnostic indicators:
  - History and clinical signs.
- Confirmatory tests:
  - Skin biopsy and stained smears of needle aspirate. Special histological stains and microbial culture to rule out differentials.
- Differential diagnoses
  - Neoplasia, cysts, amyloidosis, collagenolytic and infectious granulomata.

Treatment and management
Therapeutic approach
- Identify and treat specific cause.
- High doses of glucocorticoids: *prednisolone: 1–2 mg/kg once daily by mouth for 2–3 weeks, dexamethasone (Opticorten, Novartis) 0.1 mg/kg once daily by mouth for 2–3 weeks.*
- Prognosis:
  - Variable response to glucocorticoids.

Bites and stings

- Nettles, wasps, bees, biting flies, spiders and snakes.
- Signs vary according to agent, amount of venom injected, host factors.

Clinical features
- Signs:
  - Papules, wheals and plaques; variable pain and pruritus; necrosis and sloughing, anaphylaxis.

Diagnosis
- Diagnostic indicators:
  - History and clinical signs.
- Differential diagnoses:
  - Other causes of urticaria, collagenolytic granuloma, unilateral papular dermatosis, viral papular dermatitis.
  - Haematoma, abscess, cysts.
  - Poisoning.

Treatment
Therapeutic approach
- Leave alone.
- Glucocorticoids, antihistamines.
- Insect repellents.
- Prognosis:
  - Varies according to source of bite or sting and host factors.

Coat problems

The maintenance of normal coat density is dependent upon the ordered cyclic activity of hair follicles which, except in areas of hair specialisation, e.g. mane and tail, pass through a growth phase – anagen, a phase of maturation – catagen, and a third or resting phase – telogen when the mature hair is shed.

After a period of time the cycle is repeated. In certain circumstances of environmental or nutritional stress or a disease process, telogen hair loss becomes synchronised and abnormal hair loss occurs. This is referred to as telogen effluvium, an event which may only be observed several months after the stimulus for its onset.

Conversely, hair loss during the growth phase – anagen effluvium – may be precipitated by more severe disease processes and some forms of medication, and may be seen within a short time of the stressful stimulus.

ALOPECIA

Definition
- Loss of hair.
- Total loss of hair affecting a normally hirsute area.
- A decrease in the number of hairs or hairs shorter than normal (this may be termed hypotrichosis).

Aetiology
- Congenital.
- Acquired.

Congenital alopecia

- Rarely if ever recorded in the horse.

Acquired alopecia

Virtually any inflammatory disease of skin will precipitate hair loss. Many of these are considered elsewhere. Examples are given below.

- Parasitic infestation: chorioptic mange, pediculosis, larval nematode dermatitis (*Pelodera strongyloides*, *Strongyloides westeri*), onchocerciasis, ticks.
- Immunological reactions: *Culicoides* hypersensitivity, cutaneous lupus erythematosus, atopy, chronic eosinophilic enteritis/dermatitis, systemic granulomatous disease, alopecia areata.
- Drug reactions.
- Contact dermatitis (Figure 6.1).
- Infections: dermatophilosis, dermatophytosis.
- Neoplasia.
- Functional disorders – seborrhoea.
- Toxicoses: heavy metal poisoning, selenium.

Toxicoses

- Crusting and scaling are also prominent signs in addition to alopecia in chemical toxicoses.

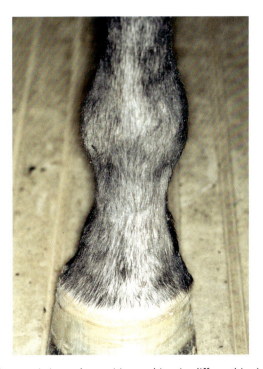

Figure 6.1   Contact irritant dermatitis resulting in diffuse thinning of the hair-coat and scaling on the distal limb after application of multiple topical therapies. Note also depigmentation of the hoof wall.

Selenium toxicosis

Clinical features
- Selenium toxicosis can result from the ingestion of grasses and cereal grains containing excessive selenium due to high soil content of selenium or the presence of selenium concentrating plants. It has also occurred with wrongly formulated feed additives.
- Occasionally concentrate feeds may be over-supplemented with selenium. Feed concentrations should not exceed 5 ppm.
- Cutaneous changes are more likely to be seen in chronic toxicity.
- Signs:
  - Whilst a rough, dry haircoat with some skin scaling is seen, the predominant signs are coronary band inflammation, hoof changes, and accompanying lameness and progressive loss of mane, tail and fetlock hair (Figures 6.2 and 6.3).
  - Generalised alopecia may develop.
  - Systemic signs may occur and include lethargy, weight loss and, ultimately, death.

Diagnosis
- History, clinical examination.
  - Selenium levels in blood, hoof and hair. Toxic tissue concentrations of selenium are typically 1–4 ppm in blood, 11–45 ppm in hair and 8–20 ppm in hoof. Selenium may also be found in the urine.
- Differentials: heavy metal toxicity.

Treatment
- There is no specific treatment for chronic selenosis.

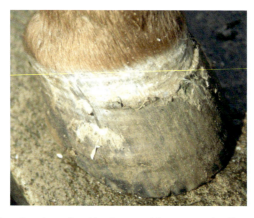

Figure 6.2 Chronic selenosis with abnormal horn growth affecting the hoof wall and shedding of the surface layers of keratin. (Courtesy of S. C. Shaw.)

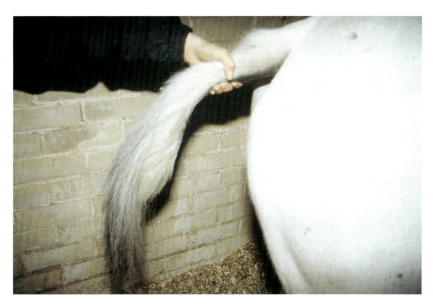

Figure 6.3   Chronic selenosis. Diffuse loss of hair from the tail ('rat tail'). (Courtesy of S. C. Shaw.)

- Change diet to reduce intake.
- *Five ppm inorganic arsenic added to drinking water.*
- *Diet high in sulphur containing amino acids, e.g. methionine supplements 2–3 g daily.*
- Recovery is prolonged and euthanasia may be indicated in animals with severe hoof deformities (Traub-Dargatz and Hamar, 1986).

Arsenic toxicosis

Clinical features
- Now a rare condition.
- Cutaneous absorption of arsenic causes irritation, drying and fissuring of the skin.
- Signs:
  - Hair loss, typically over the mane and tail is seen, although on occasions a hirsute appearance results.
  - Scaling and greasiness, and sometimes ulceration.

Diagnosis
- Based on history, clinical signs and renal or hepatic arsenic concentrations >10 ppm.
- Differentials: selenosis, mercury and other toxicoses, Cushing's disease, malnutrition.

Treatment
- *D-penicillamine at a dose of 11 mg/kg by mouth every day for 7–10 days* and removal of the source of arsenic.
- Alternative choices of therapy are:
  - *Sodium thiosulphate (10–30 g intravenously then 20–60 g by mouth every 6 h for 3–4 days).*
  - *Dimercaprol (3–5 mg/kg intramuscularly every 6 h for 2 days then twice daily for 8 days).*

Mercury toxicosis

Clinical features
- Ingestion of grain treated with organic mercurial substances, such as antifungals, may result in chronic mercury poisoning.
- Topical mercury-containing skin dressings may be licked off and/or absorbed percutaneously.
- Signs:
  - Chronic mercury poisoning results in progressive generalised alopecia and exfoliation, without hoof involvement.
  - Systemic signs include gastroenteritis, weight loss and lameness.

Diagnosis
- Mercury is concentrated in the kidneys and chronic poisoning may be confirmed post-mortem by tissue concentration > 100 ppm.

Treatment
- The source of mercury must be identified and removed.
- *Sodium thiosulphate and dimercaprol are recommended for treatment (see dose rates above) and potassium iodide 4 g by mouth daily for 10–14 days is reported to be of benefit.*

Equine alopecia areata

Clinical features
- A rare cell-mediated autoimmune skin disease.
- T lymphocytes infiltrate around and invade the hair bulb and matrix.
- Signs:
  - Appearance of non-scaling, circumscribed areas of alopecia (Figure 6.4), which may be bilaterally symmetrical.
  - Thinning of mane and tail hair.
  - Possibility of leukotrichia and/or hoof deformity.
  - Intermittent periods of remission and recrudescence may occur.
- Differentials: other non-inflammatory alopecias.

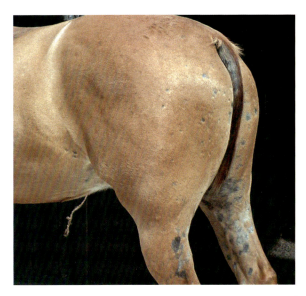

Figure 6.4   Alopecia areata. Generalised patchy alopecia with marked alopecia of the tail.

Diagnosis
- Histopathology of biopsy specimen from the edge of a new lesion to confirm lymphocytic attack on anagen-phase hair bulbs.

Treatment
- Corticosteroids are of uncertain efficacy. Systemic, topical or intra-lesional.
  - Prednisolone: 1 mg/kg once daily for 2–3 weeks.
  - *Dexamethasone (Opticorten, Novartis): 0.1 mg/kg once daily for 2–3 weeks.*
  - *Methylprednisolone acetate: 5–10 mg per lesion. Repeat after 2 weeks if necessary.*
  - *Triamcinolone acetonide: 3–5 mg per lesion. No more than 20 mg per horse. Repeat after 2 weeks if necessary.*

Prognosis
- Treatment may be ineffectual.
- Spontaneous hair growth is likely, initially with white hair.

Cushing's disease

Clinical features
- Hyperadrenocorticism (HAC) is most commonly found in cases with hyperplasia or adenoma of the pars intermedia of the pituitary.

- Hypersecretion of pro-opiomelanocortin (POMC) due to loss of inhibition by dopamine, which is insensitive to corticosteroid negative feedback, is thought to be responsible. Processing of POMC results in the production of melanocyte-stimulating hormone, corticotrophin-like intermediate lobe peptide, beta-lipotropin, beta-endorphins and adrenocorticotropic hormone (ACTH).
- A condition of older horses and ponies.
- Skin signs:
  - The most striking feature is hirsutism and affected animals show an excessively long, dense and curly haircoat that is not shed normally (Figure 6.5).
  - The mane and tail are usually unaffected.
  - Skin is often moist and greasy.
  - Skin and other infections may be present.
- Systemic signs:
  - Lethargy, pot-bellied appearance, muscle wasting, polydipsia and polyuria, infections.
  - Bulging supraorbital fat pads may be present.
- Laminitis may be a serious complication.

Diagnosis
- The commonest laboratory abnormalities are elevated alkaline phosphatase and hyperglycaemia.

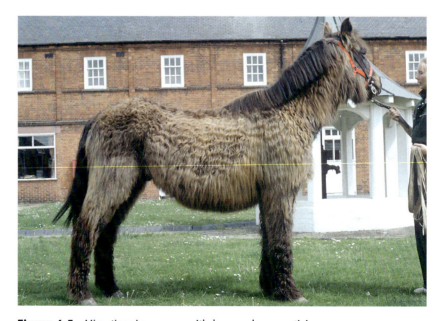

Figure 6.5   Hirsutism in a pony with hyperadrenocorticism.

- Intercurrent diabetes mellitus is common.
- Relative neutrophilia and lymphopenia may also be found together with elevation of liver enzymes, but are less consistent findings compared with the dog.
- Plasma insulin concentrations are commonly elevated – a useful screening test but not a specific indicator of the disease.
- Measurement of the level of endogenous ACTH in a single blood sample is a very sensitive test for equine pars intermedia adenoma, but presents practical problems due to the rapid lability of the hormone. Refer to your laboratory for test protocol and normal values.
- Dynamic hormone tests:
    - A variety of tests has been employed to confirm the diagnosis.
    - The ACTH and thyrotropin-releasing hormone (TRH) stimulation tests are insensitive and not specific.
    - The dexamethasone suppression test is considered to be the best test because of high sensitivity and specificity. Although there have been concerns about inducing laminitis, an association has not been shown at the recommended dose.
    - After injection of 40 μg/kg dexamethasone intramuscularly normal horses show suppression of cortisol to <30 nmol/l lasting up to 24 h.
    - Horses with HAC may show suppression of basal cortisol values, but this is short-lived and affected animals do not show suppression at 20–24 h.
    - An overnight protocol offering relatively convenient sampling times, with suggested sampling times of 5 p.m., 8 a.m. and noon (0, 15 and 19 h), has been described.
- A combined dexamethasone and TRH stimulation test is currently thought to be the most sensitive method of diagnosis.
    - Dexamethasone (40 μg/kg) is injected intravenously or intramuscularly after taking a basal blood sample.
    - A second blood sample is taken 3 h later.
    - Immediately inject 1.1 mg of TRH (Protirelin, Cambridge Laboratories) intravenously, slowly over a period of a minute.
    - Take two further blood samples 30 min and 19–21 h later.
    - Submit blood samples for cortisol analysis.
- Both healthy horses and horses with HAC show initial suppression of basal cortisol concentrations, but affected horses show stimulation of cortisol after TRH administration; whereas normal horses continue to show suppression below basal values 24 h after dexamethasone injection.

Treatment

- Many animals will respond to treatment with pergolide, a dopaminergic agonist which interferes with peptide secretion by the pituitary tumour, possibly by restoring dopaminergic inhibition of secretion of POMC peptides from the pars intermedia.
  - *The recommended dose rate of 0.01 mg/kg daily by mouth may be associated with anorexia and depression, and beneficial responses are often obtained at lower doses; 0.002 mg/kg daily by mouth is commonly used.*
- *Bromocriptine mesylate (0.02 mg/kg intramuscularly twice daily) has been used successfully;* it is poorly absorbed by mouth.
- *Cyproheptadine (Periactin), a serotonin antagonist which probably acts by interfering with ACTH secretion, may also be beneficial.*
  - *Initial dose rates of 0.15–0.25 mg/kg by mouth daily are recommended reducing to alternate day therapy after 3 months.*
- Treatment with either of these drugs is expensive and often prohibitive.
- *Trilostane, an inhibitor of adrenal steroidogenesis has been shown to be beneficial; a dose of 1 mg/kg administered once daily in the evening is suggested.*
- Affected animals are often debilitated and require a high plane of nutrition. Laminitis may develop suddenly and often necessitates euthanasia.

Further reading: *See* Beech (1999).

Pigmentary disorders

Melanin production is a complex process which is:

- probably determined genetically;
- under hormonal control via the hypophysis.

HYPOPIGMENTATION – GENETIC OR ACQUIRED

- Albinism
  - Leukoderma (absence of skin pigment).
  - Leukotrichia (absence of hair pigment).

Albinism – lethal white foal disease

- The classic albino (white with pink eyes) does not occur in the horse.
- Generalised but incomplete albinism (white with pigmented irides) is inherited as an autosomal dominant trait, in the heterozygous state a quarter of all matings produce non-viable foals.
- In mating two Overo paint horses affected by a similar, but autosomal, recessive trait produce foals with albinism and congenital defects of the intestinal tract.

Leukoderma and leukotrichia

Clinical features

- Aetiology and pathogenesis: in many cases this is unclear, the following may play a part.
  - Genetics.
  - Trauma – physical, chemical, inflammatory disease.
  - Endocrine disorders and dermatoses that feature hydropic deeneration of basal cells, e.g. autoimmune disease, lupus erythematosus.
  - Neurological disorders.

- Signs:
  - Depigmentation of hair alone, leukotrichia.
  - Depigmentation of skin but not hair, leukoderma.
  - Depigmentation of skin and hair.

Arabian fading syndrome

- Also known as: Arabian pinky syndrome, Juvenile Arabian leuko-derma.

Clinical features
- A depigmentation disorder affecting 1–2-year-old horses of the Arab breed of either sex, rarely seen in older animals or horses of other breeds.
- No specific cause has been determined but, since it is seen to occur in animals of particular blood lines, genetic factors seem the more likely aetiology.
- Signs:
  - Progressive development of depigmentation over several months of the eyelids, periocular skin, muzzle and nares, perineum anus and vulva, ventral skin of the base of the tail and skin of the inguinal region.
  - No evidence of any other disease.
  - The depigmentation may be permanent, may resolve and the skin repigment, or there may be phases of depigmentation and repigmentation.

Diagnosis
- History:
  - The occurrence in a young horse of the Arab breed should suggest the diagnosis of Juvenile Arabian leukoderma.
  - Most common depigmentation disease of horses.
  - Depigmentation in an older horse would require the ruling out of diseases such as lupus erythematosus.

Treatment
- Many treatments have been offered, e.g. dietary supplementation with vitamins and minerals, no conclusive evidence of their value has been shown.
- The strong evidence for a genetic aetiology suggests a guarded prognosis and no treatment.

OTHER PIGMENTARY CHANGES CONSIDERED TO BE GENETIC IN AETIOLOGY

Appaloosa coat coloration

Clinical features
- The full white hair component of the coat of this breed develops post-natally by a process of progressive depigmentation in patches, thought to be genetically determined.
- Coat greying.
- Change of coat colour by greying has been considered to be the effect of mutant genes.

Reticulated leukotrichia

Clinical features
- Depigmentation of hair with no associated leukoderma.
- Particularly affects quarter horses, although it has been thought to occur in Thoroughbreds and Standardbreds.
- Aetiology: unclear, but because of the significant breed incidence it is thought to be genetic.
- Signs:
  - Mainly in young horses, yearlings.
  - Non-painful crusted dermatitis having a linear distribution and following a cross-hatched pattern.
  - The lesions extend from the withers to tail.
  - Resolution of lesions is followed by growth of permanently white hair.

Treatment
- None effective.

Spotted leukotrichia

Clinical features
- Acquired spots of white hair. Arab horses appear predisposed.
- Aetiology: unclear, possibly initiated by trauma.
- Signs:
  - Multiple areas of white hair, with or without leukoderma.
  - Symmetrical distribution over the hindquarters and thorax.
  - No evidence of pruritus or pain.
- Treatment:
  - There is no treatment for this condition.

HYPOPIGMENTATION FOLLOWING INFLAMMATION

- Inflammatory changes in the skin commonly result in associated areas of loss of pigment, often permanent, for which there are many causes, some examples of which follow.

Infective conditions

Parasitic

- Trypanosomiasis – *Trypanosoma equiperdum* infection ('Dourine'): genital infection of males and females, ulceration of genitalia with depigmentation, urticarial wheals on the neck, shoulders and back.
- Onchocerciasis, ventral midline dermatitis.
- *Parafilaria multipapillosa* infestation, seasonal larval migration through the skin.

Bacterial and fungal

- Deep infection leading to ulceration through the skin surface.

Viral

- Aural plaques – papovavirus infection. *Simulium* flies may act as vectors.
- Coital exanthema – EHV-3 infection: papular vesicular and pustular lesions on the genitals of mare and stallion. Oral, nostril and lip lesions are occasionally seen. Healed lesions show permanent depigmentation.

Non-infective conditions

Hypersensitivity

- *Culicoides* hypersensitivity (sweet itch).

Autoimmune diseases

- Cutaneous lupus erythematosus.
- Equine erythema multiforme.
- Hyperaesthetic leukotrichia.

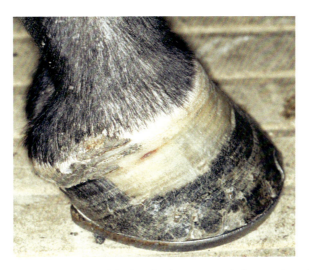

Figure 7.1   Depigmentation of the hoof subsequent to inflammation of the coronary band due to contact irritant reaction after multiple topical therapies applied to the distal limb.

Disorders of keratinisation

- Linear keratosis.
  - Areas of crusting, hair loss and subsequent depigmentation.

Physical and chemical agents

- Cold branding, cryosurgery, burns.
- Trauma:
  - wounds from ill fitting harness, etc., plaster casts, rope burns, deep skin wounds. Flank depigmentation in stallions – self-trauma.
- Chemical agents (Figure 7.1):
  - Blisters, rubber toxicity, primary irritant contact dermatitis.

Hyperpigmentation

- A common non-diagnostic change seen in some chronic inflammatory, hormonal, developmental or neoplastic disorders of animals (Jubb et al., 1985).
- Hyperpigmentation is rare in horses, with the exception of melanocytic tumours of grey horses, multicentric melanoma.

Melanotrichia

- Small areas of dark hairs occasionally occur at sites of inflammatory reaction.

Pastern leucocytoclastic vasculitis

See Chapter 3.

The foot and associated structures

The foot includes the hoof wall, the sole and the frog, and the coronary band including the periople (Figures 8.1 and 8.2). These structures enclose the distal part of the second phalanx and the third phalanx with its sesamoid (the navicular bone) and cartilages (the lateral cartilages).

THE HOOF WALL

The coronary matrix extends around the proximal border of the hoof, heel to heel, and from this the hoof wall grows. Associated with this is the marginal matrix, which gives rise to the periople.

The inner aspect of the wall of the hoof is folded into numerous (approximately 600) horny laminae, which interdigitate with the vascular sensitive laminae.

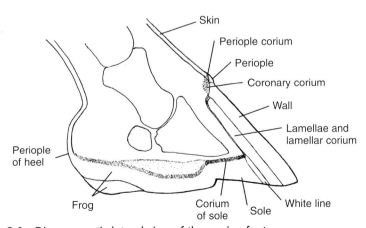

Figure 8.1 Diagrammatic lateral view of the equine foot.

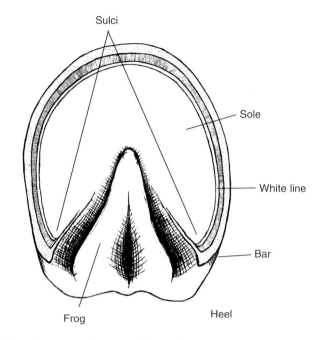

Sulci

Sole

White line

Bar

Frog

Heel

Figure 8.2 Diagrammatic view of the undersurface of the equine foot.

The sensitive laminae overlie the third phalanx and provide nourishment to the inner wall of the hoof. The horny sole is similarly nourished. The hoof may vary in its pigmentation; melanin follows the line of the horn tubules. In horses with non-pigmented hooves, injury, causing extravasation of blood, may lead to incorporation of haemoglobin into the hoof wall and discoloration.

Hoof growth

- Hoof horn in mature horses grows at approximately a quarter to three-eighths of an inch (c. 0.64–0.95 cm) per month and requires trimming every 4–6 weeks. Replacement of the wall takes between 9 and 12 months.

The periople

- The periople is an area of modified coronary band tissue in which production of soft, non-pigmented keratohyalin of varnish-like consistency extends around the hoof and also downwards, preventing excess moisture loss from the wall of the hoof.

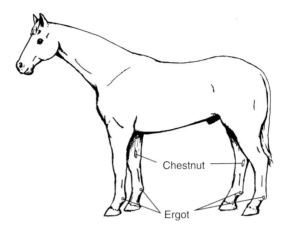

Figure 8.3   Vestigial horny structures of the equine limbs.

The sole

- The sole is composed of hard keratin, often with a flaking surface, and is usually either concave or flat. Its junction with the hoof wall forms the 'white line', which provides an anatomical guide for nail placement when shoeing.

The frog

- This is a V-shaped, soft, pliable, elastic structure extending from the heel to the centre of the sole. It has no hard hoof horn.

Other horny structures

- The vestigial horny structures of the limbs of the horse should not be ignored (Figure 8.3). Their inclusion in the examination of the foot is important in the differential diagnosis of hoof disorders.
- The ergots are considered to be vestiges of the second and fourth digits and chestnuts remnants of the first digit.

EXAMINATION OF THE FOOT

- By visual inspection and palpation.

Visual inspection

- Examine the stance of the foot.
- Look for more wear on one side than the other related to the conformation of the limb.
- Uneven wear and weight bearing induces cracks.
- Note appearance of hoof rings. Annular rings are normal. Disruption of the annular conformation may be indicative of disease.
- Be aware of the normal differences in the shape between fore and hind feet.

Manual examination

- Enables the texture of the coronary band to be determined. Normally it is slightly papillomatous.
- Problems of the coronary band may include traumatic wounds, discoloration (bruising) and specific diseases (Figure 8.4 and 8.5), such as pemphigus coronitis, selenium toxicity, superficial necrolytic dermatitis (hepatocutaneous syndrome).
- Identify abnormalities of the horn, e.g. cracks, changes in pigmentation (Figure 8.6).
- Feel the temperature of the foot.
- Assess for presence of pain, by use of hoof testers and digital pressure. Observe gait for any lameness or functional impairment.

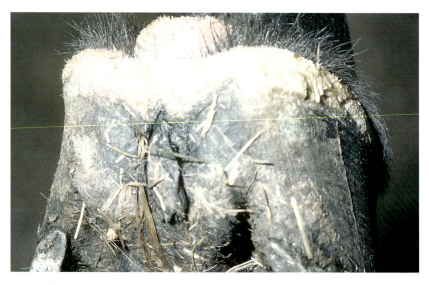

Figure 8.4   Chronic coronitis with frog damage in a show hack.

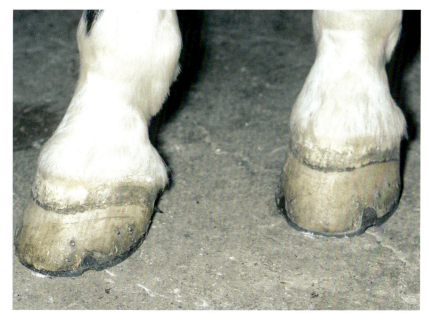

Figure 8.5   Hoof ring formation in a 10-year-old show jumper caused by chronic coronitis.

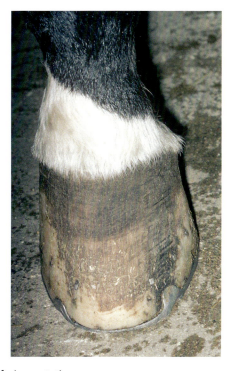

Figure 8.6   Hoof pigmentation.

DISORDERS OF THE FOOT

Genetic defects

- Flat feet. Absence of normal concave sole.
- Thin walls and soles. Walls break away. Shoeing is difficult.

Treatment
- Good farriery and stable management.

Aplasia cutis

- Also known as: epitheliogenesis imperfecta – hoof slough.

ACQUIRED DISORDERS OF THE HOOF

Hoof rings

Clinical features
- Variation in production of wall keratin.
- Aetiology: dietary changes; laminitis; coronitis; systemic disease.
- Signs: a series of rings of keratin overgrowth or reduction around the wall, the most pronounced being due to laminitis.

Treatment
- Correct underlying causes.
- Careful farriery.

Cracks

Clinical features
- Wall, heel, toe, quarter and sole cracks.
- Aetiology: bad foot care; traumatic damage; systemic disease.
- Signs: vertical or transverse cracking of the hoof wall, deep cracks may involve the sensitive laminae and cause lameness.

Treatment
- Special farriery procedures.

Keratoma

Clinical features
- Tumour of the hoof wall.

Treatment
• Surgical ablation, resection of hoof wall; possibly cryosurgery.

Coronary band dystrophy

Clinical features
• An uncommon specific entity in the horse in which there is a defect in cornification.
• Aetiology: unknown; this is a diagnosis of exclusion, made after eliminating other possible causes.
• Affected animals have been mature horses; large or heavy breeds appear predisposed.
• Signs:
  – All or part of the coronary bands of all feet affected.
  – Lesions of proliferation and exudation of coronary band tissue followed by hyperkeratosis (Figure 8.7). Ergots and chestnuts may be affected.
  – Severe cases show lameness.
  – Histological changes are not well documented; abnormalities involve the epidermis with papillary hyperplasia and papillary squirting (spongiosis) over tips of dermal papillae, and overlying hyperkeratosis which may be parakeratotic.

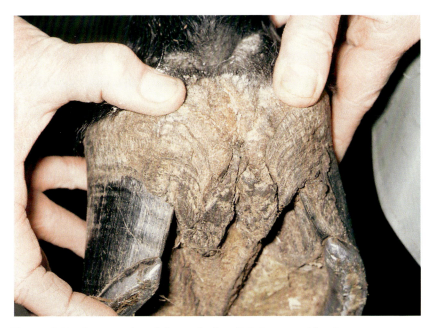

Figure 8.7 Coronary band dystrophy in a Belgian warmblood.

Treatment
- Symptomatic.

Differential diagnosis of coronary band disease
- Trauma – initiated by pruritus due to parasitism or accidental.
- Pemphigus foliaceus. May be the only site of lesions, coronary band separation (*see* Autoimmune diseases in Chapter 7).
- Epidermolysis bullosa. Hoof separation.
- Chronic eosinophilic enteritis. Weight loss, exudative and ulcerative coronitis.
- Superficial necrolytic dermatitis (hepatocutaneous syndrome). Bacterial infection of the liver. Weight loss, coronary band separation.
- Selenosis. Coronary band separation with associated loss of hair of mane and tail.
- Extension to coronary band of infective organisms: dermatophilosis, foot abscess (pricked foot); chorioptic mange causing self-trauma.
- Seborrhoea. In severe generalised disease there is accompanying coronary band dystrophy with poor hoof conformation – boxy hooves.
- Sarcoid.

THE FROG

- Anticoncussion and antislipping action: to remain healthy and well developed must have contact with the ground.

Thrush

Clinical features
- Necrotic condition of the horn sulci extending to involve the whole of the frog.
- Aetiology: Poor management; standing in unhygienic conditions; soiled wet bedding, mud; failure to clean out hoofs regularly.
- Infection with necrosis organisms, *Fusobacterium necrophorum* (Figure 8.8).
- Signs:
  - More prevalent in hind feet than fore.
  - Can occur in any one or more feet.
  - Distinctive foul necrotic odour when foot is examined.
  - Affected sulcus has a thick, black, moist, malodorous discharge.
  - Probing may show the sulcus to be deeper than normal.

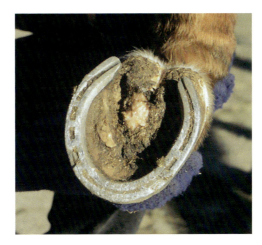

Figure 8.8   Anaerobic infection of the hoof.

Diagnosis
- Absence of lameness in most cases.
- Black discharge and malodour.

Treatment
- Improve stable management.
- Clean dry standing.
- Regular foot hygiene.
- Initial debridement and daily application of antimicrobial solution until tissue returns to normality. *Chlorhexidine and miconazole shampoo (Malaseb, Leo) can be used. Severe cases may need systemic antibiotic therapy, e.g. procaine penicillin at 15 mg/kg twice daily for 5 days.*
- Astringents may also be useful.
- May require special shoeing.

Canker

- Similar to thrush but predominantly affects hind feet, particularly in draft horses.
- A disease associated with poor management. Predisposition when horses are kept in wet conditions.
- Maceration and infection of the heel, bars and frog sulci occurs.

Treatment
- Astringent dressings.
- Debridement.
- Treat severe cases as for thrush.

Frog overgrowth

Clinical features
- Aetiology unknown.
- Signs: no gross anatomical abnormality; rapid and excessive growth of frog epithelium.
- Excess frog thickness without adequate wear is detrimental to foot conformation.

Diagnosis
- On history, clinical findings.

Treatment
- One of the only reasons for judicious paring of excess tissue by the farrier.

NEOPLASIA OF THE FROG

Fibroma

Clinical features
- Signs:
  - Occurs at similar site to thrush; malodorous; black necrotic tissue in sulcus.

Diagnosis
- Signs, history.

Treatment
- Surgical ablation.

NECROSIS

- Aetiology: ischaemia.

THE SOLE

Bruised sole

Clinical features
- Aetiology: injury due to – stones, hard dry terrain, bad shoeing, laminitis.
- Signs:
    - Vary with severity of injury.
    - Blood streaking in solar keratin.
    - Bleeding under sole.
    - Exudation of serum at coronary band.
    - Underrunning infection.

Treatment
- Relieve
- Farriery; pressure.
- Treat infection.

Therapy in equine dermatology

AVAILABILITY OF VETERINARY MEDICINES FOR EQUINE PATIENTS

Background

- The horse is classified in the European Union (EU) as a minor food-producing species.
- If a medicinal product is to be used in food-producing animals then it must have had a maximum residue limit (MRL), in addition to market authorisation (product licence), by 1 January 2000.

Current position (1999)

- The UK government considers that if a horse is not destined for human consumption then MRLs are not required. The French and Irish authorities have the same view.
- Where no authorised product for a condition exists, in particular to avoid causing unacceptable suffering to the animal concerned, the veterinary surgeon may administer another product (Council Directive 81/851/EEC).
- The 'Cascade' (Medicines [Restrictions on the Administration of Veterinary Medicinal Products] Regulations 1994: SI 199413142) states that only veterinary medicinal products licensed for use in food-producing animals may be used for food-producing animals. There are exceptions to this rule, but veterinary surgeons who feel that circumstances compel them to use a medicine not covered by the available legislation are advised to contact the Veterinary Medicines Directorate (VMD). The Regulations will be interpreted in the light of how a competent and professional veterinary surgeon would reasonably act in a particular set of circumstances. No suffering that

can be treated without placing consumers at risk is acceptable (AMELIA8).
- The British Equine Veterinary Association (BEVA) has issued guidelines on the use of medicines in equidae.
- Note that the bioavailability of drugs may differ in different formulations. Users should refer to product datasheets for relevant information.

Sources of drugs, topical products and instruments

Bayer plc, Animal Health Business Group, Eastern Way, Bury St Edmunds, Suffolk IP32 7AH, England. Tel: 01284 763 200.

Cambridge Laboratories, Richmond House, Brewery Court, Sandyford Road, Newcastle upon Tyne NE2 1XG, England. Tel: 0191 261 5950.

Carr & Day & Martin Ltd, Lloyds House, Alderley Road, Wilmslow, Cheshire SK9 1QT, England.

CEVA Animal Health, 7 Awberry Court, Hatters Lane, Watford, Hertfordshire WD18 8PE, England. Tel: 01923 212212.

Day Son & Hewitt Ltd, St George's Quay, Lancaster LA1 5QJ, England. Tel: 01524 381 821.

Fort Dodge Animal Health, Flanders Road, Hedge End, Southampton SO30 4QH, England. Tel: 01489 781 711.

Hortichem Ltd, 1b Mills Way, Boscombe Down Business Park, Amesbury, Wiltshire SP4 7RX, England.

Intervet UK Ltd, Walton Manor, Walton, Milton Keynes, Buckinghamshire MK7 7AJ, England. Tel: 01908 665 050.

Janssen Animal Health, PO Box 79, Saunderton, High Wycombe, Buckinghamshire HP14 4HJ, England. Tel: 01494 567 555.

Janssen-Cilag Ltd, PO Box 79, Saunderton, High Wycombe, Buckinghamshire HP14 4HJ, England. Tel: 01494 567 567.

JHC Healthcare Ltd, The Maltings, Bridge Street, Hitchin, Hertfordshire SG5 2DE, England. Tel: 01462 432 533.

Kalium Products Ltd, West Court, Morton Bagot, Studley, Warwickshire B80 7EL, England. Tel: 01527 857 870.

Leo Laboratories Ltd, Longwick Road, Princes Risborough, Buckinghamshire HP27 9RR, England. Tel: 01844 347 333.

Merial Animal Health Ltd, Sandringham House, Harlow Business Park, Harlow, Essex CM19 5GT, England. Tel: 01279 775 858.

Thomas Pettifer & Company Ltd, Newchurch, Romney Marsh, Kent TN29 0DZ, England. Tel: 01303 874 455.

Pfizer Animal Health, Walton Oaks, Dorking Road, Tadworth, Surrey KT20 7NS, England. Tel: 01737 331333.

Schering-Plough Animal Health, Breakspear Road South, Harefield, Uxbridge UB9 6LS, England. Tel: 01895 626 000.

Sorex Ltd, St Michaels Industrial Estate, Widnes, Cheshire WA8 8JT, England. Tel: 0151 420 7151.

Squibb, Bristol-Myers Squibb Pharmaceuticals Ltd, 141–149 Staines Road, Hounslow, Middlesex TW3 3JA, England. Tel: 020 8572 7422.

SSL International plc, Turbiton House, Oldham OL1 3HS, England. Tel: 0161 652 2222.

Vericore Veterinary Products, Novartis Animal Health UK Ltd, New Cambridge House, Littlington, Hertfordshire SG8 0SS, England. Tel: 01763 850 500.

VetPlus Ltd, Dock Road, Lytham, Lancs FY8 5AQ, England. Tel: 01253 667422.

Virbac Ltd, Woolpit Business Park, Windmill Avenue, Woolpit, Bury St Edmunds, Suffolk IP30 9UP, England. Tel: 01359 243 243.

References and further reading

Booth, T.M. and Wattret, A. (2000) Stifle abscess in a pony associated with *Myco-bacterium smegmatis*. *Veterinary Record*, 147: 452–454.

Beech, J. (1999) Diseases of the pituitary gland. In *Equine Medicine and Surgery*, Vol. II (5th edition). St Louis, MO: Mosby.

Couto, C.G. (1994) Lymphoma in the horse. In *Proceedings of the 12th Annual Forum of the American College of Veterinary Internal Medicine*, San Francisco, p. 865.

Curtis, C.F. (1999) Pilot study to investigate the efficacy of a 1% selenium sulphide shampoo in the treatment of chorioptic mange. *The Veterinary Record*, 144: 674–675.

Fadok, V. (1998) Differential diagnosis of equine pruritus: parasites as allergens and irritants. *ESVD Workshop on Equine Dermatology Course Notes.* Newmarket, pp. 6–11.

Goodrich L., Gerber, H., Marti, E. and Antczak, D. F. (1998) Equine Sarcoids. *Veterinary Clinics of North America: Equine Practice*, 14: 607–623.

Gortel, K. (1998) Equine parasitic hypersensitivity. *Equine Practice*, 20: 14–16.

Herd, R.P. and Donham, J.C. (1988) Efficacy of ivermectin against Onchocerca cervicalis microfilarial dermatitis in horses. *American Journal of Veterinary Residents*, 44: 1102–1105.

Hillyer, M.H., Taylor, F.G.R., Mair, T.S., Murphy, D., Watson, T.D.G. and Love, S. (1992) Diagnosis of hyperadrenocorticism in the horse. *Equine Veterinary Education*, 4: 131–134.

Jacobs, D.E. (1986) *A Colour Atlas of Equine Parasites.* London: Baillière Tindall.

Johnson, P. (1998) Dermatologic tumours (excluding sarcoids). *Veterinary Clinics of North America*, 14: 625–657.

Jubb, K.V.F., Kennedy, P.C. and Palmer, N. (1985) *Pathology of the Domestic Animals*, Vol. 1 (3rd edition). London: Academic Press, p. 415.

Knottenbelt, D.C. and Pascoe, R.R. (1994) *Color Atlas of Diseases and Disorders of the Horse.* London: Wolfe Publishing.

Knottenbelt, D.C. and Kelly, D.F. (2000) The diagnosis and treatment of periorbital sarcoid in the horse: 445 cases from 1974 to 1999. *Veterinary Ophthalmology*, 3 (2–3): 169–191.

Littlewood, J.D. (2000) Chorioptic mange: successful treatment of a case with fipronil. *Equine Veterinary Education*, 12: 144–146.

Littlewood, J. D. (1999) Control of ectoparasites in horses. *In Practice*, 21: 418–424.

Littlewood, J.D., Rose, J.F. and Paterson, S. (1995) Oral ivermectin paste for treatment of chorioptic mange in horses. *Veterinary Record*, 137: 661–663.

Littlewood, J.D., Whitwell, K.E. and Day, M.J. (1995) Equine cutaneous lymphoma: a case report. *Veterinary Dermatology*, 6: 105–111.

Lyons, E.T., Drudge, J.H. and Tolliver, S.C. (1988) Verification of ineffectual activity of ivermectin against adult *Onchocerca* spp. in ligamentum nuchae in horses. *American Journal of Veterinary Research*, 49: 983–985.

McCalla, T.L., Moore, C.P. and Collier, L.L. (1992) Immunotherapy of periocular squamous cell carcinoma with metastasis in a pony. *Journal of the American Veterinary Medical Association*, 200: 1678–1681.

Monahan, C.M., Chapman, M.R., French, D.D. and Klei, T.R. (1995) Efficacy of moxidectin oral gel against *Onchocerca cervicalis* microfilariae. *Journal of Parasitology*, 91: 117–118.

Mozos, E., Novales, M., Sierra, M.A. and Millan, J. (1991) Focal hypopigmentation in horses resembling Arabian Fading Syndrome. *Equine Veterinary Education*, 3: 122–125.

Newton, S.A. (2000) Periocular sarcoids in the horse: three cases of successful treatment. *Equine Veterinary Education*, 12: 137–143.

Ossent, P. and Lischer, C. (1997) Post-mortem examination of the hooves of cattle, horses, pigs and small ruminants under practice conditions. *In Practice*, 19: 1.

Pascoe, R.R. (1990) *A Colour Atlas of Equine Dermatology*. London: Wolfe Publishing.

Pascoe, R.R. (1981) *Equine Dermatoses*. University of Sydney Post Graduate Foundation in Veterinary Science, pp. 73–85.

Paterson, S. and Orrell, S. (1995) Treatment of biting lice (*Damalinia equi*) in horses using selenium sulphide. *Equine Veterinary Education*, 7: 304–306.

Paterson, S. (1997) Dermatophytosis in 25 horses. *Equine Veterinary Education*, 9: 171–173.

Pollitt, C.C. (1995) *Colour Atlas of the Horses Foot*. London: Mosby Wolfe.

Rosenkrantz, W.S., Griffin, C.E., Esch, R.E. and Mullens, B.A. (1998) Responses in horses to intradermal challenge of insects and environmental allergens with specific immunotherapy. In K.W. Kwochka, T.W. Willemse and C. von Tscharner (eds), *Advances in Veterinary Dermatology*, Vol. 3. Oxford: Butterworth Heinemann, pp. 191–200.

Rosenkrantz, W. (1998) Selected topics in equine dermatology: Pruritic hypersensitivities. *ESVD Workshop on Equine Dermatology Course Notes*, pp. 13–15.

Scholl, P. (1998) Moxidectin 2% equine oral gel. *Equine Practice*, 20: 19–21.

Scott, D.W. (1988) *Large Animal Dermatology*. Philadelphia: W.B. Saunders.

Stannard, A.A. and Pascoe, R.R. (1994) *ESVD Workshop on Equine Dermatology Course Notes*. London: European Society of Veterinary Dermatology.

Stashak, T.S. (1987) *Adam's Lameness in Horses (4th edition)*. Philadelphia: Lea & Febiger, pp. 532–541.

Theon, A. (1998) Intralesional and topical chemotherapy and immunotherapy. *Veterinary Clinics of North America: Equine Practice*, 14: 659–671.

Thomsett, L.R. (1991) Pigmentation and pigmentary disorders of the equine skin. *Equine Veterinary Education*, 3: 130–135.

Traub-Dargatz, J.L. and Hamar, D.W. (1986) Selenium toxicity in horses. *Compendium on Continuing Education for the Practising Veterinarian*, 8: 771–776.

von Tscharner, C., Kunkle, G. and Yager, J. (2000) Stannard's illustrated equine dermatology notes. *Veterinary Dermatology*, 3: 161–223.

Index

Note: page numbers in *italics* refer to figures

abscess 31, *63*, 74, 77
  differential diagnoses 64, 65, 80,
    94, 95, 99
acantholytic keratinocytes 37
acanthoma, papillary 70
acaricides 13, 82
Acarus 14
acepromazine 17
Actinobacillus 75
Actinomyces (actinomycosis) 75, 78
adrenocorticotrophic hormone
    (ACTH) 106, 107
albinism 109
allergens, avoidance 21, 23
allergies 15, 22, 52
alopecia 4, 100–5
  atopy 20, 101
  cicatricial 39
  Culicoides hypersensitivity *19*, 101
  cutaneous lupus erythematosus
    39, 101
  demodicosis 81, *82*
  dermatophilosis *32, 33, 34*, 101
  exfoliative eosinophilic dermatitis
    and stomatitis/enteritis 44
  fly irritation 17
  generalised granulomatous
    disease 42
  greasy heels syndrome 44
  iodism 41
  louse infestation 9, *10*
  mange 13, 101
  pemphigus foliaceus *36*, 37
  photosensitisation *60*
  pressure sores 56
  seborrhoea 26, 101
  sunburn *58*
  toxicoses 41, 101, 102, 103–4
  Trichophyton 28
  tuberculosis 77
  viral papular dermatitis 71
alopecia areata 68, 101, 104–5
Alternaria alternata 16, 79
amphotericin B 79, 80
amyloidosis, cutaneous 85, 88, 91,
    92, 96, 98
anaemia, louse infestation 9

anagen/anagen effluvium 100
analgesia 17, 56
anaphylaxis 81, 99
androgens 85
angio-oedema 23–4, 52
anorexia in pemphigus foliaceus 37
anti-inflammatory treatment 17, 20,
    21, 46
antibiotics 35, 48, 52, *53*, 56, 73, 114
anticonvulsants, drug eruptions 52
antihistamines 20, 21, 99
antipruritic therapy 20
aplasia cutis 120
    see also epitheliogenesis
        imperfecta
Appaloosa breed 35, 111
Arab horses 39, 54
Arabian fading syndrome 110
arsenic, organic 103
arsenic toxicosis 103–4
arsenic trioxide 68
aspirin, drug eruptions 52
atopy 19, 20–2, 101
aural plaques 70–1
autoantibodies 37, 50
autoimmune disease 104, 109, 112
axillary nodular necrosis 90–1
azathioprine 38

bacille Calmette–Guérin (BCG)
    vaccination 68, 87
bacteria/bacterial infections 4, 6,
    30–3, *34*, 35, 72–7
  hoof 122, *123*
  hypopigmentation 112
  pastern folliculitis 114
  secondary infection 11, 48, 49
bacteriology, nodular disease 63
bandages, support 73
bees 17
Belgian Draft breed 54
benzyl benzoate topical cream 20
benzylpenicillin 73, 74
betamethasone 85–6
biopsy 6, 7–8, 24, 39, 45
bites 98–9
black fly 17, 70, 112

bleomycin 68
blisters 113
botryomycosis *16*, 75, *76*
brachytherapy 87
bromocriptine mesylate 108
bruising 64, 65
  foot 118, 125
bullous pemphigoid 44, 49, 50
burns 55–6, 113
bursitis 65

calcinosis circumscripta 65, 90, 93,
    96
callus formation 56
canker 123
carboplatin 68
ceftiofur 32, 73, 76
cellulitis 31, 33, 73
chestnuts 117, 121
chlorambucil 86
chlorhexidine 29, 31, 35
  and miconazole shampoo 29, 32,
    35, 46, 123
chloroxylenol 26, 27, 32
Chorioptes 11, 12, 45
chromomycosis 79
chrysotherapy for pemphigus
    foliaceus 38
cimetidine 85
cintronellol 20
cisplatin 68, 85, 87
clinical examination 2–3
Clostridium myositis 74
coat
  brushings 5
  problems 100–8
  see also alopecia; leukotrichia
Coatex Medicated shampoo *see*
    chloroxylenol
coital exanthema 48–9, 50, 112
cold branding 113
collagen 54, 55
  degeneration *see* granuloma,
    collagenolytic
complement C3 39, 62
corns 56, 57
coronary band 37, 118, *119, 120–3*

coronitis, pemphigus 118
corticosteroids 39
    alopecia areata 105
    bullous pemphigoid 50
    cutaneous habronemiasis 48
    drug eruptions 52
    erythema multiforme 51
    generalised granulomatous
        disease 43
    greasy heels syndrome 46
    onchocercal dermatitis 16
    pastern leucocytoclastic vasculitis
        62
    pemphigus foliaceus 38
    photosensitisation treatment 61
    see also named drugs
Corynebacterium pseudotuberculosis
    74, 75
creosote, contact dermatitis 22
crusting and scaling lesions 4, 6, 18,
    19, 22, 25–46, 101
    environmental causes 40–1
    immune-mediated 35–40
    infectious causes 27–30
    uncertain aetiology 42–6
cryosurgery 68, 70, 87, 113, 121
cryotherapy 85
Culicoides (midges) 17
    hypersensitivity 15, 18–20, 101,
        112
Curvularia geniculata 77
Cushing's disease 103, 105–8
cyclophosphamide 86
cypermethrin 10, 14, 20
cyproheptadine 108
cysts 93–5
    differential diagnoses 64, 74, 81,
        92, 95, 98, 99
cytology, direct smears 6
cytosine arabinoside 86
cytotoxic agents 70

Damalinia equi 10
defecation problems 84
Demodex 81
demodicosis 5, 6, 68, 72, 81–2
depigmentation 39, *58, 101,* 110–13
Dermanyssus gallinae 14
dermatitis
    contact 19, 20, 22–3, 33, 101
        irritant 40–1, 45, 113
    exfoliative eosinophilic and
        stomatitis or enteritis 43–4, 45
    hyperplastic of ear 70
    idiopathic pastern 45
    larval nematodes 16, 101
    onchocercal 15–16
    proliferative 11
    subepidermal vesicular 50
    superficial 20, 118, 122
    viral papular 70, 71–2, 90, 93, 99
Dermatophilus (dermatophilosis) *16,*
    32–3, *34,* 35, 45, 101
    differential diagnoses 28–9, 31, 37,
        44–5, 68, 72, 122
dermatophytes 4, 5, 6, *16*
dermatophytosis 4, 27–30, 101
    differential diagnoses 31, 33, 37,
        44–5, 68, 72, 90, 93

dermatosis *36, 57, 58,* 90, 92–3, 99
dermo-epidermal junction 50
dexamethasone 21, 24
    alopecia areata 105
    collagenolytic granuloma 90
    cutaneous lymphoma 85
    nodular panniculitis 98
    pemphigus foliaceus 38
    unilateral papular dermatosis 93
dexamethasone suppression test 107
diagnosis 3–9
    differential *2, 3*
diet 22, 103
DiffQuick stain 4, 6
digital pressure 118
dimercaprol 104
discoid lupus erythematosus (DLE)
    38–9
diuretics, drug eruptions 52
DNA papovavirus 70
Dourine 112
Drechslera spicifera 16, 79
drug eruptions 50, 52, *53,* 59, 101
dust, reaction to 20
dystocia 84

ectoparasites *see* parasites/parasitic
    infestations
Ehlers–Danlos syndrome 54–5
electrocautery of sarcoid 68
enilconazole 29
enrofloxacin 32, 73, 76
enteritis, chronic eosinophilic 101,
    122
eosinophilic granuloma *see*
    granuloma, collagenolytic
eosinophils 37
epidermolysis bullosa 54, 122
epitheliogenesis imperfecta 53–4,
    120
equine herpes virus (EHV) 3 48, 49,
    50, 112
ergots 117, 121
erythema *32,* 39, 44, *58,* 59
    multiforme 40, 50, 51, 112
ethyl lactate 32
excoriated lesions 6
exudate, impression smears 63

fatty acids, essential 22
fetlock, horse pox 49
fever, pemphigus foliaceus 37
fibroma 68, 85
fibrosarcoma 68
fipronil 12, 14
fistula 94, 95
flies 17, 47, 81
    see also black fly
flumethrin 12
5-fluorouracil 68, 87
folliculitis *16,* 27, 68, *82*
    pastern 31, 33, 45, 114
    staphylococcal 29, 30–2, 72, 90, 93
    streptococcal 30–2
food 20, 22, 103
foot 3, 115–25
    disorders 4, 120–5
    examination 117–18, *119*
    frog 117, 122–4

sole 116, 117, 125
    see also greasy heels syndrome;
        hoof
foreign body 94, 95
fungal granuloma 76
fungal infections *16,* 27–30, 41, 75,
    76, 77–80, 112
fungi
    cultures 45, 63
    direct smears 6
furunculosis *16,* 30–2, 90, 93
Fusobacterium necrophorum 122, *123*

gait 118
genital infections 49
gentamicin 73
Giemsa stain 4, 6
girth gall 57
girth itch 27
glucocorticoids
    axillary nodular necrosis 91
    bites/stings 99
    collagenolytic granuloma 90
    cutaneous lymphoma 85
    exfoliative eosinophilic dermatitis
        and stomatitis or enteritis 44
    mastocytosis 92
    nodular panniculitis 98 ·
    topical 23, 26
    unilateral papular dermatosis 93
    see also named drugs
gold therapy for pemphigus
    foliaceus 38
Gram's stain 4, 6
granulation tissue, exuberant 48, 68,
    76, 86, 97
granuloma 81
    collagenolytic 79, 88–90
        differential diagnoses 81–2, 85,
            88, 91, 92–3, 96, 98–9
    fungal 76
    infectious 48, 68, 82, 91, 96, 97, 98
granulomatous disease 37, 42–3, 44,
    101
greasy heels syndrome 11, 31, 32,
    33, 44–6, 114
griseofulvin 29

Habronema (habronemiasis) 47–8, 68,
    76, 86, 97
Haematobia (horn fly) 17
haematoma 64, 65, 74, 99
Haematopinus asini 10
hair 4, 100
    see also alopecia; coat; leukotrichia
harvest mites, larval stages 5
health status, general 2–3
heavy metal toxicosis 101, 102,
    103–4
heels *see* greasy heels syndrome
helminths 15–16, 47–8
hepatocutaneous syndrome
    118, 122
Heracleum mantegazzianum (giant
    hogweed) 60
herbage collection/examination 8
hernia 65
hirsutism 106
hogweed, giant 60

hoof 115–17
  boxy 122
  canker 123
  cracks 120
  pigmentation 116, 118, *119*
  ring formation *119, 120*
  slough 120
  thrush 122–3
  wall *101,* 115–16
hoof testers 118
horn fly 17
horse fly 17
horsepox 45, 49–50
houseflies 47
husbandry 1
hydrocortisone 39
hydroxyzine hydrochloride 20, 21, 24
hyperadrenocortism 105–8
hyperkeratosis 56
hyperpigmentation *10,* 20, 113–14
hypersensitivity 45, 47, 52, 112
  see also Culicoides (midges), hypersensitivity
Hypoderma (hypodermiasis) 80–1, 82, 90
hypopigmentation 109–13
hypotrichosis 100

imidazole foggers 30
immune reactions 101
immune stimulation 68
immunoglobulin G (IgG) 39, 62
immunoglobulin M (IgM) 39
immunosuppression 43, 50
immunotherapy 22, 86
impression smears of exudate 63
infections 16, 33, 56, 101, 112
  nodular or swollen lesions 66, *67,* 68–80
  see also bacteria/bacterial infections; fungal infections; viral infections
injection abscess *63,* 74
injury *see* trauma
insect attack 17, 98–9
  see also black fly; flies
insect bite hypersensitivity 15, 20, 89
  see also Culicoides (midges), hypersensitivity
insect repellants 17
insecticides 10, 17, 20
intradermal tests 20, *21*
intravenous fluid therapy for burns 56
iodides 78, 79, 80, 104
iodism 41, 79
itraconazole 79, 80
ivermectin 52, 82
  oral paste 11, 12, 15, 16, 48

joint capsule, enlarged 65

keratinisation disorders 112
keratinocytes, acantholytic 37
keratoma 120–2
keratosis, linear 112
ketoconazole 79, 80

lameness 118
laminitis 106, 108
laser therapy 69, 87
leukoderma 39, 109–11
leukotrichia 40, 109–11, 112
lice 5, 9–11, 15, 101
lichenification, atopy 20
ligatures, sarcoid 68
light oil 20
limb
  cellulitis 31, 33
  oedema 33
linear keratosis 112
local anaesthetics, drug eruptions 52
lupus erythematosus, cutaneous 38–40, 50, 101, 109, 112
  see also systemic lupus erythematosus (SLE)
lymphadenopathy 77, *87*
lymphangitis, ulcerative 74–5
lymphoma, cutaneous 85–6
lymphosarcoma 91

Mackenzie brush technique 5, 29
maculopapular rash 22
malignancy 83
malnutrition 103
mane
  rubbing 18, *19*
  seborrhoea 25–6
mange
  chorioptic 5, 11–12, 45, 101, 122
  psoroptic/sarcoptic 12–13
mastocytosis 85, 88, 91–2, 96
megoestrol acetate 86
melanocytic tumours 84, 113
melanoma 83–5, 113
melanomatosis, dermal 84
melanotrichia 113
mercury toxicosis 103, 104
methionine supplements 103
methotrexate 85
methylene blue, systemic photosensitisation 59
methylprednisolone 20, 90, 91, 92, 105
miconazole 29, 32, 35
microorganisms 4, 16
  see also bacteria/bacterial infections; fungal infections; viral infections
Microsporum 5, 16, 27, 29
midges *see Culicoides* (midges)
mites 5, 11–14, 20, 45
  see also mange
molluscum contagiosum, equine 70, 72
mosquitoes 17
moulds 20
  see also fungal infections
moxidectin gel 15, 16
mud fever 32, 44
  see also greasy heels syndrome
Musca domestica (housefly) 47
mycetoma 74, 75–8, 79, 80, 88, 92
Mycobacterium (mycobacterial infections) 75, 77
mycoses *see* fungal infections
myositis, clostridial 74

natamycin 29
navicular bone 115
necrobiosis, nodular *see* granuloma, collagenolytic
needle aspirates 6–7, 63
nematodes, larval 16, 101
neoplasia 83–7, 101, 124
  differential diagnoses
    abscess 74
    axillary nodular necrosis 91
    bacterial mycetoma 76
    bursitis 65
    calcinosis circumscripta 96
    collagenolytic granuloma 90
    conchal cyst 95
    cutaneous amyloidosis 88
    cyst 94
    demodicosis 82
    dermoid cyst 95
    hernia 65
    hypodermiasis 81
    injury 64
    mastocytosis 92
    nodular panniculitis 98
    sporotrichosis 80
    unilateral papular dermatosis 93
Neotrombicular autumnalis 13–14
neurofibroma/neurofibrosarcoma 68
neutrophils 37
nevus, melanocytic 84
Nikolsky's sign 53, 54
nits 10
Nocardia (nocardiosis) 75
nodular or swollen lesions 4, *7,* 63–99
  cysts 93–5
  immune-mediated causes 87–8
  infectious causes 66, *67,* 68–80
  neoplasia 83–7
  parasitic infestations 80–2
  physical conditions 64–5
non-steroidal anti-inflammatory drugs (NSAIDs) 52, 61, 73

oatmeal, colloidal 20
oedema 33, 37, 44, 59
onchocerciasis 68, 101, 112
Oxyuris equi 4, 15, 19, 20

panniculitis 85, 98
papillary acanthoma 70
papillomatosis 68, 69–70, 72
papovavirus 112
papules 20, *23*
Parafilaria multipapillosa 112
parasites/parasitic infestations 4, 5, 9–15, 20, 80–2, 101
  aberrant 47
  hypopigmentation 112
pastern
  folliculitis 31, 33, 45, 114
  greasy heels syndrome 44, *45*
  horse pox 49
  leucocytoclastic vasculitis 33, 61–2
  mud fever 32
Paxcutol shampoo 26, 27
pediculosis *see* lice

Pelodera strongyloides 16, 101
pemphigus coronitis 118
pemphigus foliaceus 29, 35–8, 44, 122
D-penicillamine 104
penicillins 52, *53*
    see also benzylpenicillin; procaine penicillin
pergolide 108
periople 115, 116
permethrin 10, 14, 20
phaeohyphomycosis 79, 80
phenothiazines 52, 59
phenylbutazone drug eruption 52
photoallergy 58, 59
photodynamic agents 58, 59, 60
photosensitisation 33, 45, 57, 58–61, 62
phototoxicity 58
phylloerythrin 59
pigmentary lesions 4, 109–14
    see also depigmentation
piroctone olamine 26, 27, 32
podophyllin 68
poisoning 99
    see also toxicoses
pollen, reaction to 20
potassium iodide 104
potassium monopersulphate sprays 30
povidone iodine 31
pox virus 45, 49–50, 71, 72
prednisolone 20, 21, 23, 24, 86
    alopecia areata 105
    collagenolytic granuloma 90
    cutaneous lupus erythematosus 40
    erythema multiforme 51
    generalised granulomatous disease 43
    mastocytosis 92
    nodular panniculitis 98
    pastern leucocytoclastic vasculitis 62
    pemphigus foliaceus 38
    unilateral papular dermatosis 93
pressure sores 56–7, 91
pro-opiomelanocortin (POMC) 106
procaine penicillin 32, 73, 75
progestagens 85
protozoa, direct smears 6
pruritis/pruritic lesions 4, 25, 44
    contagious conditions 9–16
    non-contagious 17–24
Pseudoallescheria boydii 77
Pseudomonas mycetoma 75
pseudomycetoma, fungal/bacterial 78
Psoroptes 13
pustular lesions 6
Pyemotes 14
pyoderma 31, 81
pyrethrins 10, 14
pyrethroids, synthetic 17

Quarter horse 26, 54, 55

radiation therapy 69, 87, 92
radiofrequency hyperthermia 69
ragwort 61
rain scald 32
rhinopneumonitis vaccine 40
rubber toxicity 113
rupture 65
rye grass, perennial 59

saddle sores 56
St John's wort 59
sarcoid 66, *67*, 68–9
    differential diagnoses 48, 70, 85, 86, 97, 122
    fibroblastic 48, 66, *67*, 68, 86, 97
sarcoid cream 68
sarcoidosis, equine 42–3
Sarcoptes scabiei 13
scaling lesions 4, 11, 20, *58*, 59
    see also crusting and scaling lesions
scalp brush 5
scirrhous cord 65
Sebomild P shampoo *see* piroctone olamine
seborrhoea 25–7, 37, 101, 122
sedation 8, 17, 56
selenium sulphide shampoo 11, 12, 26, 27
selenium toxicosis 101, 102–3, 118, 122
self-trauma 4, 113, 122
shampoo 20, 35
    miconazole and chlorhexidine 29, 32, 35, 46, 123
    selenium sulphide 11, 12, 26, 27
Simulium (black fly) 17, 70, 112
sit-fasts 56, 57
skin grafting for burns 56
skin scrapings 5–6, 12, 14
smears, direct 6
sodium aurothiomalate 38
sodium thiosulphate 104
Sporothrix schenckii 80
sporotrichosis 75, 79–80
squamous cell carcinoma 48, 68, 85, 86–7, 97
squamous papilloma 70
stable fly 17, 47
stallions, flank depigmentation 113
staphylococci 16, 73, 74, 75, *76*
    see also folliculitis, staphylococcal
Staphylococcus aureus 114
stings 98–9
Stomoxys (stable fly) 17, 47
streptococci 16, 30–2
Strongyloides westeri 101
stud crud 26
sulphadiazine *see* trimethoprim and sulphadiazine
sulphonamides 52, 59
sulphur 103
summer sores 47–8
sunburn 57, *58*
sunlight avoidance 39, 61, 62
sunscreens 39
suppliers 128–9

swabs 6
sweet itch *see Culicoides* (midges), hypersensitivity
systemic lupus erythematosus (SLE) 38–9, 44
    see also lupus erythematosus, cutaneous

T lymphocytes 104
Tabanus (horse fly) 17
tail 15, 18, 25–6, 31, *78*, *103*
tape strippings 4
telogen/telogen effluvium 100
tetracyclines 59
thiazides 59
Thoroughbred racehorses 73
thrush 122–3
thyrotrophin-releasing hormone (TRH) stimulation test 107
ticks 101
toxicoses 41, 101–4, 118, 122
tracheotomy 88
trauma 4, 64, 113, 118, 122
triamcinolone acetonide 90, 92, 105
Trichophyton 16, 27, *28*, 29, 30
trilostane 108
trimethoprim and sulphadiazine 32, 73, 76
trombiculidiasis 45
trypanosomiasis 112
tuberculosis 77

ulcerative and erosive lesions 4
    congenital/hereditary causes 53–5
    contagious causes 47–50
    dermatoses 57–62
    environmental causes 55–7
    immune-mediated causes 50–2, 53
ulcerative lymphangitis 74–5
ultraviolet radiation 57
urticaria 10, 20, 21, 23–4, 52, 64, 99

vaccines 30, 40, 68, 87
vaccinia virus-infected autologous tumour cell 86
vasculitis 33, 44, 45, 61–2
vesicular stomatitis 50
vetch, hairy 42
veterinary medicines 126–7
vincristine 86
viral infections 48–50, 66, *67*, 68–72, 112
    see also dermatitis, viral papular
vitiligo *see* leukoderma
vulva, horse pox 49

warble fly 81
warts, aural flat 70
wasps 17
Werneckiella (Damalinia) equi 10
white foal disease, lethal 109
worming routine 15
wounds 113

yeasts 4